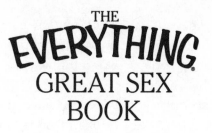

THE EVERYTHING GREAT SEX BOOK

Dear Reader,

I am thrilled that you have chosen this book. I hope it will serve as a useful tool in your journey toward a happier and more fulfilling sex life.

By improving your intimate relationships, you improve your life overall. You have already taken an important first step. By seeking out resources such as this book, you are making the effort to ensure your sexual relationships are the best they can be. While great sex often happens spontaneously, that doesn't mean you don't need to practice or prepare. A little legwork beforehand can greatly improve your bedroom experiences. As a bonus, your partner will appreciate your efforts to help both of you achieve more satisfying sexual experiences.

Everyone's bedroom tastes and desires are different, so you won't find any "right" or "wrong" answers here. Think of this book as a starting point, from which you can go off on sorts of creative—and exciting—directions.

Bobbi Dempsey

WITHDRAWN

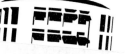

Welcome to the EVERYTHING Series!

These handy, accessible books give you all you need to tackle a difficult project, gain a new hobby, comprehend a fascinating topic, prepare for an exam, or even brush up on something you learned back in school but have since forgotten.

You can choose to read an *Everything*® book from cover to cover or just pick out the information you want from our four useful boxes: e-questions, e-facts, e-alerts, and e-ssentials.

We give you everything you need to know on the subject, but throw in a lot of fun stuff along the way, too.

We now have more than 400 *Everything*® books in print, spanning such wide-ranging categories as weddings, pregnancy, cooking, music instruction, foreign language, crafts, pets, New Age, and so much more. When you're done reading them all, you can finally say you know *Everything*®!

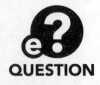

QUESTION

Answers to
common questions

FACT

Important snippets
of information

ALERT

Urgent
warnings

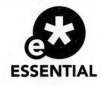

ESSENTIAL

Quick
handy tips

PUBLISHER Karen Cooper

DIRECTOR OF ACQUISITIONS AND INNOVATION Paula Munier

MANAGING EDITOR, EVERYTHING® SERIES Lisa Laing

COPY CHIEF Casey Ebert

ACQUISITIONS EDITOR Katrina Schroeder

ASSOCIATE DEVELOPMENT EDITOR Elizabeth Kassab

SENIOR DEVELOPMENT EDITOR Brett Palana-Shanahan

EDITORIAL ASSISTANT Hillary Thompson

EVERYTHING® SERIES COVER DESIGNER Erin Alexander

LAYOUT DESIGNERS Colleen Cunningham, Elisabeth Lariviere, Ashley Vierra, Denise Wallace

Visit the entire Everything® series at *www.everything.com*

THE EVERYTHING®

GREAT SEX BOOK

2nd Edition

Your complete guide to passion,
pleasure, and intimacy

Bobbi Dempsey

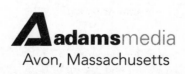

Avon, Massachusetts

This book is dedicated to all the passionate
romantics out there.

An Everything® Series Book.
Everything® and everything.com® are registered trademarks of F+W Media, Inc.

Published by Adams Media, a division of F+W Media, Inc.
57 Littlefield Street, Avon, MA 02322 U.S.A.
www.adamsmedia.com

ISBN 10: 1-4405-0148-3
ISBN 13: 978-1-4405-0148-7

Printed in the United States of America.

10 9 8 7 6 5 4 3 2 1

Library of Congress Cataloging-in-Publication Data
is available from the publisher.

This publication is designed to provide accurate and authoritative information with regard to the subject matter covered. It is sold with the understanding that the publisher is not engaged in rendering legal, accounting, or other professional advice. If legal advice or other expert assistance is required, the services of a competent professional person should be sought.

—From a *Declaration of Principles* jointly adopted by a Committee of the American Bar Association and a Committee of Publishers and Associations

Many of the designations used by manufacturers and sellers to distinguish their products are claimed as trademarks. Where those designations appear in this book and Adams Media was aware of a trademark claim, the designations have been printed with initial capital letters.

Interior illustrations by Eric Andrews

This book is available at quantity discounts for bulk purchases.
For information, please call 1-800-289-0963.

Contents

Acknowledgments

The author wishes to thank Gina Panettieri, who made this project possible, and Katrina Schroeder, who made sure it was a positive experience.

Top 10 Benefits
of Great Sex

1. Physical health. Statistics show that you will live longer and stay in better shape if you are having great sex. Learning proper breathing techniques and doing your Kegel exercises will add quality of life as well.

2. Mental health. Great sex contributes to a better sense of personal growth, strengthens the connection you have with your partner, and has a calming effect in your life.

3. Emotional health. Happiness and satisfaction with life come with having a great sexual connection.

4. Knowing that you are a great lover will make you glow.

5. Your lover will greatly appreciate the bliss in your relationship.

6. Very cost-effective marriage therapy. Practicing the communication techniques included in this book will greatly enhance your relationship skills.

7. Long, luxurious, sexy, creative, affordable dates. You and your partner will learn to cherish your time together and make every moment count.

8. Ongoing development of your creativity muscles. The more you engage in great sex, the more you think up new, interesting positions, techniques, and places in which to have it.

9. Knowledge advice, and ideas to share with your friends. You can pass on tips to your friends to help them improve their relationships as well.

10. You'll have a lot of fun!

Introduction

AS GEORGE MICHAEL ONCE sang, "Sex is natural, sex is fun." While both statements may be true, it may not always feel that way. Yes, sex is a natural, biological process as old as mankind, but for many people—especially those who are self-conscious in the bedroom—sex (good sex, at least) may not seem to come naturally. And if you are worried, anxious, self-conscious, or otherwise distracted, sex probably won't be much fun, either.

The good news is, great sex isn't an impossible feat. In fact, it may be much more attainable than you may think. It may take a little bit of effort and perhaps a little practice (which will be fun, I promise!) but before you know it, your sex life will be better than you ever dreamed possible.

The truth is, you probably already have the basic ingredients for a terrific sexual experience: desire, passion, primal urges, and a willing partner. Most likely, you are letting yourself get way too hung up on technique (or your perceived lack thereof) and how you insert Tab A into Slot B. Fortunately, that's stuff you can easily learn, if you have the motivation and dedication. And, since you've made the effort to pick up this book, I'm assuming you are indeed eager to learn. That's half the battle.

Exploring and learning about our sexual nature comes easily to some people and seems challenging to many others. We aren't taught much about sex unless we were lucky enough to have parents who weren't afraid to talk about it. Young people learn about sex from their peers or from experimentation. The older a person gets before he has experienced some kind of sexual encounter, the more ill-equipped that person will feel upon actually entering a sexual relationship.

When we feel well informed, practiced, and excited about sex, it becomes an awesome experience. We are born with all the right equipment for sex. What we need is a sort of an "owner's manual"—a guide to help us learn, give us ideas with which to experiment, and supply the guidelines to let us know that we are on the right track.

Every couple and every sexual encounter a couple has is unique. It may not feel that way to you right now, but, as you begin to learn more about your sexual nature, you will begin to observe the differences each time you make love. By doing this you will have a basis from which to expand even further. Becoming conscious—but not self-conscious—while having sex is the key to having each separate experience feel new, exciting, and creative.

Each one of us is responsible for our own sexual happiness. It isn't our lover's responsibility, though it is wonderful if we feel partnered with someone who wants to have sexual happiness, too. *The Everything® Great Sex Book, 2nd Edition* is designed with the goal of giving you every tool necessary to have a complete, satisfying, expansive sexual and sensual experience.

The topics included in this book make it a complete resource for relationships, sexuality, and intimacy. It will help you put a lifetime of fun into your intimate life. From male and female anatomy lessons and erotic sexual positions to effective communication techniques and ideas from the Kama Sutra, it will enlighten and inform you. This book has been designed to be useful again and again, allowing you to delve deep into the information you need for a lifetime of great sex.

You won't find a more complete book than this on any bookstore shelf. It is a guide that will inform you for many years to come and provide the insight and knowledge you need for a future of great sex. A long life, a healthy life, a happy life, and a great sex life all go together!

CHAPTER 1

What Is Great Sex?

For some people, just being able to have any sex at all is enough of a treat to be considered "great." For others, great sex must transport the partners to a state of blissful oneness of body, mind, and spirit. A lot of people think great sex is any sex that brings a deep sense of satisfaction and fulfillment to both partners. Take some time to think about what great sex means to you.

Why Can't Sex Be Simple?

Why all the fussing and fretting about sex? Why can't sex be simple? Well, it could be, if the human mind didn't have the tendency to want to be in control of the human body. Most people have been taught to trust their minds and ignore messages from their bodies. All the major institutions of socialization—churches, schools, businesses, and even family—teach you to control your impulses so you don't get into trouble or embarrass yourself or someone else.

As you get older, the mind begins to exert yet another type of control. You learn that it's not safe to do things that might offend or upset people. So you learn how to behave to get other peoples' approval. By the time you have your first adult sexual experience, the whole area of sexual relationships has gotten pretty complicated. You have learned numerous strategies for controlling yourself and for manipulating the opinions and feelings of others. This situation does not bode well for enjoying a lifetime of great sex.

ALERT

Worry is one of the common killers of great sex. Humans worry about everything. Most of the time it is a futile exercise that keeps us from diving deeply into intimacy. Don't allow needless and excessive worrying to prevent you from sharing enjoyable intimate experiences with your partner.

In spite of this early conditioning, the innate desire for satisfying intimate relationships remains strong. It just needs to be encouraged, and it will re-emerge. This book can help you get back in touch with your own essential nature and reclaim your own life force. With a little patience and practice, your sex life can be transformed from something mundane or problematic to something wonderful and fun.

Not Just Maintenance Sex

Great sex is not just any sex at all; it is certainly not what may be called maintenance sex. Maintenance sex is what some people do most of the time when having sex—where partners perform sex more as a routine than as a conscious, intentional celebration of their love.

Maintenance sex is entirely acceptable, but it is not to be confused with sex that is *really great*. Maintenance sex generally involves some degree of compromise—a step or two down from one's ideal. Perhaps only one partner is in the mood, and the other complies. One of the partners may be trying to appease the other. Or maybe, at times, one or both partners simply want to do the minimum to maintain their sense of being sexually connected.

By contrast, great sex is usually transformative and healing for the partners. Partners feel loved and cherished, and all seems right with the world. Great sex can help partners transcend their separateness from each other. They both become part of something larger—a spiritual connection that puts them in touch with the oneness of all creation. Great sex may not happen automatically. But it can be learned. To have great sex requires knowledge, skill, patience, time—and practice!

And Much, Much More

After having great sex, people often report that petty ego concerns and personality conflicts seem unimportant. Competitive ideas about feminine and masculine roles or responsibilities tend to fade. The stresses of looking good, being in control, feeling separate, or being on guard disappear. Great sex involves honesty, trust, letting go, merging, and just being.

Great sex is not so much about technique as it is about presence. The most technically skilled lover is nothing without an open, trusting presence and attention to her or his partner. Learning new positions, techniques, and tricks is only a vehicle for experiencing each other's presence in new ways.

Great sex is a type of intimate communication. It is one of the most important ways in which you, as a human being, share who you are with your partner. Really great sex is like melting or dissolving into a universal state of oneness.

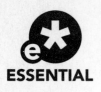

Think of great sex as a bonding experience. Sharing your vulnerability with your partner creates a special connection that can help you deal with the not-so-fun parts of the relationship. Great sex can benefit all areas of your relationship, both in and out of the bedroom.

Who's Doing It (and When and How)

When it comes to sex, it seems like it is only natural—and often irresistible—to compare ourselves to other people. We all imagine that everyone else is doing it better (or more often) than we are, and that we simply don't measure up. So it might be helpful to consider some statistics. But just remember: Great sex is more about quality than quantity. Just because someone else is having sex more often doesn't mean they are having good sex more often. Think about it: Would you rather have blah, ho-hum sex every night of the week, or incredible mind-blowing sex once or twice a week? Exactly.

So here are some stats you might find interesting:

- According to a 2008 survey by *Health* magazine, 64 percent of respondents have sex at least once a week. That's similar to the findings of a *Redbook* survey, where 60 percent reported having sex at least once or twice a week (5 percent claimed to be having sex on a daily basis). A majority of the *Redbook* respondents said they wish they were having sex more often.
- One-third of the *Health* respondents named the missionary position as their favorite, with "woman on top" ranked a close second. By contrast, a *Cosmopolitan* survey of men found they loved the woman-on-top position best.
- As for solo action, 27 percent of the *Health* group said they masturbate at least once a week, while another 25 percent said they pleasure themselves at least once a month (although some said they only masturbate when their partners are unavailable).

What It Really Takes

There are only a handful of key elements to having great sex: curiosity, openness of heart and mind, the willingness to try new things and learn, and a willing partner or partners. Within that handful, though, there is a vast array of possibilities for self-expression. The skills and techniques in this book are meant to enhance your own unique self-expression—this isn't a one-size-fits-all cookbook.

Sex as a Metaphor for Life

One could say that how you "do" sex is a metaphor for how you "do" life. Your sexual relationships reflect the same habitual patterns and survival strategies, learned as a child, that you exhibit in other areas of your life—except these patterns are often even more pronounced in the sexual arena. If you want to change one or more of the habitual ways you react to things, sex is a good place to start.

FACT

In a recent Tantra.com online survey, 2,400 people responded to this statement: Making love to my partner is more than sexual release; it's an experience of union with what I think of as spirit or our souls meeting. Of those surveyed, 40 percent responded "frequently," 45 percent responded "occasionally," and 15 percent responded "never."

If you have trouble asking for what you want, for example, sex is a good learning laboratory. It's an area of life that is concrete. The feedback you get from your actions is clear: You either ask or you don't—and you either get what you asked for or you don't. With such clear and unequivocal feedback, learning is more likely to occur. And when you learn a basic life skill such as self-expression, this learning will easily transfer to the other areas of your life. It is the premise of this book that a life of consistently great sex is possible and that it can be fun to train yourself to get there.

Beyond Your Wildest Dreams

Learning new sexual and sensual techniques can bring you more than simple physical pleasure. You may also find yourself feeling a sense of ongoing unity with your lover. Healing can occur not only with respect to your sexuality, but also in your faith and trust in life, your emotions, and your health. Your overall self-confidence will grow as you learn to communicate and understand each other better.

Sexual healing has vast ramifications. Whenever you experience healing of past blocks or inhibitions, you tend to become happier, more generous, and more self-trusting. And you tend to pass this happiness on to those around you. When you feel loved, understood, sexually fulfilled, and connected, you become much more powerful as a human being. This is especially important for those women and men who were taught to suppress or deny their natural sexuality.

Basic Assumptions of This Book

Every book or author has a point of view, a set of basic assumptions underlying the principles and practices the author writes about. We all bring our personal history, education, and experiences to the table when we speak or write. The first and foremost assumption in this book is that life is a precious gift that each person is entrusted with at birth. You are given a body, a mind, and a set of resources and limitations to work with. It is up to you to use what you have to make the most of what you have been given. The purpose of life is self-realization—to realize your true nature and potential.

How Is That Related to Sex?

Sex is a vital aspect of life that can result in both new life and in a profound experience of oneness between partners. As such, it holds the potential for allowing you to partake in the divine nature of creativity, which includes both procreation (birthing a child) and co-creation (birthing new ideas, products, services, or works of art). Sex can also be a great source of pleasure, joy, and fun!

The experiences of a lifetime are the curriculum that allow you to learn about your true nature and develop your innate gifts and talents. If life is a school, Sex and Intimate Relationships is the advanced course. If you welcome these lessons as opportunities to learn about yourself and expand your capacity to deal creatively with life, then you will feel happy most of the time.

ESSENTIAL

Life operates on the principle of mutual benefit. A relationship is a living system, and as such it is a good place to experience this principle. The more high-quality attention you put into your relationship, the more high-quality benefits you will derive from it.

Honesty Is a Prerequisite for Intimacy

If you want to have an intimate relationship, not a superficial one, complete honesty is necessary. If you keep secrets from your partner, you are affirming that you cannot trust that this person has your best interests at heart. If you do not trust a person in this way, ask yourself, "Why would I want to have sex with this person?" If mistrust is present, it's a good idea to be honest about this. Often, honest communication reveals your own projections, baggage, or recurrent fears held over from childhood. Expressing them honestly can allow you to get over them.

Your feelings of mistrust may reveal more about you than about your partner. This is one reason it's good to share what you feel and think—so you can discover the hidden layers of truth about yourself that may underlie your feelings about your partner. Sometimes fears about telling the truth are based on false beliefs learned in childhood. Now that you are an adult, it's time to update your beliefs about what is really safe and what is really dangerous.

Risk-Taking Leads to Confidence

If you fear doing something that you really want to do, it is usually a good idea to go ahead and take the risk. You may want to pause and honestly assess the risk before doing so, but more often than not, the risk will turn out to be more about damage to your ego than to your physical or emotional well-being. Most interpersonal risks are not life threatening. Remember that fear is not a sign to turn back but rather a sign that you are moving into unknown territory. If you take the risk and survive, which you probably will even if it doesn't turn out as you'd hoped, your confidence will grow.

You Are Responsible

You are responsible for your own experience. Whatever you feel or think about another person is a mirror of where you are. If someone does something that upsets you, you are responsible for your feelings of being upset. Likewise, when you feel satisfied with something your partner did, you are responsible for that, too. The other person does not make you happy. Likewise, he does not make you upset.

Your lover or partner is not responsible for your pleasure. You are. Learning about your own body—what you like, how you respond, and how to ask for what you want—are essential skills for great sex. Blaming your lover for not giving you orgasms or not doing it right will get you nowhere. Empower yourself to learn the skills to ask for what you want in a straightforward, loving, and truthful way.

Pleasure Is Your Birthright

Our bodies are pleasure instruments that need to be played to stay in tune. Why would nature have given you erogenous zones if you weren't meant to do something with them? By learning to play that instrument, you train your body to receive great amounts of pleasure. When you know how to receive, your view of the world changes. You begin to see the world as benevolent and trustworthy. Then you give that energy back to the people in your life.

The Adventure Before You

This book has been designed to be both a resource guide and an inspiration to you. It covers a vast array of information on anatomy, intimacy, relationships, latest discoveries, and fun sexual and sensual techniques. Good relationships and great sex go together, so you'll find both topics covered here.

You'll see how old attitudes from your past can block pleasure and honest self-expression. You'll have the opportunity for self-assessment so you can get an up-to-date view of yourself instead of operating from an outdated self-image. You will be guided to understand where you are now and to develop a plan for where you want to go. You'll have better tools to decide what you want out of life.

ESSENTIAL

Transforming some of your sexual experiences into sacred rituals will help your bodies remember the event. This will cause you to look forward to more sexual and sensual experiences, which will then begin a feedback loop that becomes self-reinforcing. Life will look fresh and alive.

Sex is one of life's most wonderful gifts—whether, at any given moment, it is wonderful for you or not. It can be a great teacher. Although it can be fraught with anxiety and stress, it can be easy, fun, and relaxing. If you want to discover your highest potential for great sex, trust yourself and don't be afraid to try something new. If you do, one thing is for sure—your capacity for aliveness and pleasure will grow. At the very least, this book could lead to some of the cheapest and best dates you've ever had in your life. Use it well and enjoy.

Sexual Myths, Misconceptions, and Mistakes

A well-informed lover is often a better lover. By the same token, a lack of information or a lot of misinformation can sabotage your love life. Let's sort out the sexual facts and fallacies and attack some common sexual misconceptions.

Sex Is Totally Automatic

Many people seem to think that we're born with a gene that tells us exactly how to make love. With sex, the raw passion and animal attraction is often a natural, instinctive phenomenon. But that doesn't mean the entire process will be the same way. There are a lucky few who just seem to be born sexual dynamos. For most people, though, great sex takes practice and patience.

One Bad Experience Spells a Doomed Relationship

It may be true that you only get one chance to make a first impression, but that doesn't mean you should base an entire relationship on the first encounter. For one thing, an initial sexual encounter often occurs in the heat of the moment, perhaps under the influence of alcohol and/or other substances. In other words, one or both of you may not be at your best. Plus, many couples find that their lovemaking improves as the relationship grows and trust deepens.

Sex Shouldn't Be Work

Okay, nobody is saying sex should be like spending a twelve-hour shift working in the coal mines. But think about it: Most of us spend lots of time and energy becoming better parents, employees, homeowners, pet owners, etc. Yet we feel embarrassed about studying sex techniques. That's just silly! Your sex life is one of your most important priorities, so you should be eager to devote the same time to improving it as you would anything else in your life that's meaningful to you. Plus, this is perhaps the most fun type of work you'll ever have. Think of how much you and your partner will enjoy spending lots of time improving and perfecting your lovemaking techniques.

Once a Bad Lover, Always a Bad Lover

First of all, it can be argued that there's no such thing as a bad lover. If someone has an unimpressive technique or is hesitant or nervous in bed, it's probably because of a lack of experience, lack of self-confidence, negative sexual experience(s) in his or her past, or other issues that, in most cases, can be addressed and resolved. If you have an otherwise good relationship with your partner, but he or she doesn't quite get your blood racing in the bedroom, consider this your opportunity to be a sexual teacher and mentor. Help him or her become a better lover (in a gentle, sensitive way, of course) and you will both reap the benefits.

CHAPTER 2

History and Mythology

Relax, this is one history lesson you'll enjoy. You might find it interesting to learn about the history of sex. Knowing where you've come from can help you see where you are going. It can be instructional to look at sex and love from a historical perspective. Our biological nature, the role of religion, family structures, and the constraints of culture—all of these have affected the history of sex and love.

A Brief History of Sex and Love

Sex has been on our minds and in our loins forever—all throughout human existence. Though most of us relate to sex from our own relatively limited perspective, many varying attitudes have been present throughout history. Even today there is a wide range of acceptability when it comes to human sexuality.

At the Dawn of Civilization

Early humans didn't know that it took a man's sperm to fertilize the woman's egg to create a baby. Whether they thought the gods, spirits, or the woman herself created the baby, they didn't connect the act of sex with procreation. Family units as we know them today didn't exist, and few human societies had the monogamous relationships we now know as marriage.

By the time the world's cultures had developed writing, women's status had diminished tremendously. Men prevailed in most aspects of the culture, with a few rare exceptions.

ESSENTIAL

When you think about it, the heavens must be a romantic place, as they seem to be filled with many different deities who focus on love. Eros, the ancient Greek god of love, is equivalent to Kama, the Hindu god of love. (Kama is often depicted as a young cherub type of creature, armed with a bow and arrow, so he's very similar to our idea of Cupid.) Psyche, or Soul, is the Greek counterpart to Shakti, the supreme Hindu goddess.

Ancient India and the Kama Sutra

India and most of the Far East were essentially patriarchal societies, but women were held in higher regard than in other cultures of the times. The woman was the initiatress and the energy behind the sexual life force. In Eastern culture, sexuality achieved the status of an art form.

As a result, ancient treatises on love like the *Kama Sutra*, the *Ananga-Ranga*, and the *Ishimpo*, traditionally passed down as oral histories, were recorded in written form for future generations. But even in India and other countries of the Far East, sexuality eventually lost its sacredness and society became more sexually conservative.

Europe in the Middle Ages

After the fall of the Roman Empire and the spread of Christianity, sexuality became limited to procreation. The romantic, courtly love of the Middle Ages is well known for its purity and piety. The troubadours pined for their true love in beautiful songs but didn't do much more about it. Sex and morality were, for the first time in history, converging.

The Christian church put many dampers on the family, sex, and even having children. Strict theologians went so far as to recommend abstinence on Thursdays, in memory of Christ's arrest; on Fridays, in memory of his death; on Saturdays, in memory of the Virgin Mary; and on Sundays, in honor of the Resurrection. Mondays, Tuesdays, and Wednesdays were often religious holidays and fasts, so intercourse was banned on those days as well. Good Christians were not supposed to have sex during Lent, which lasted forty days, or on Christmas or other religious holidays and fasts. All of those restrictions meant the number of days you weren't allowed to have sex far outnumbered the days sex was permitted.

It wasn't until the mid-1600s that Europe began to transform. Within a few short years, sanitation, science, life expectancy, and the nuclear family all began to flourish.

FACT

Organized religion played a great role in the formation of one partner and one family. Great constraints were placed upon couples and society to conform to the moral imperative of the times. Our modern perception of sex as sinful arose during this time.

The Victorian Age and Beyond

The age of modesty, imposed leisure, and protection from the dangers of the world put middle-class women into a long period of forced subservience during the Victorian Age. Menstruation was considered a disability and sexual desire was not appropriate for a virtuous woman. Men were the superior gender. And yet, during this time of restraint, prostitution flourished, both in Europe and America. Men would go to prostitutes so as not to bother their delicate wives. This was a time of misguided virtuous behavior.

The advent of World War I brought women into the modern world with work opportunities and a bit more independence. By 1920, women in Britain, Australia, New Zealand, and America could vote. They were beginning to join the work force and they were gaining new freedom.

Sexual Liberation

This was the start of the feminist movement and the beginning of a new sexual liberation for women. Through the struggles of the last century women have come to a fresh, modern perspective. Today, both men and women are finding their way through the maze of new relationship and gender problems and opportunities that are characteristic of modern society.

Sex and Intimacy Today

In many ways, the world seems to have turned a corner in recent years. People today are more comfortable openly discussing sex and sexual issues. The print media has played a big part in contributing to the comfort of talking about sex. Major magazines, both men's and women's, compete at the newsstand with headlines that boast the latest techniques and secrets. Talk shows dealing with relationships and sex are among the hottest on TV.

Thanks to modern technology, you can access sexual information and erotic material via your computer in the privacy of your own home. On the other hand, technology has also allowed us (for better or worse) to let down our guard and open up more quickly to people we barely know. Computers are blamed for a host of relationship problems, from fueling online porn habits or obsessions to facilitating casual hookups and extramarital affairs.

Then there's the fast pace of our modern lives. Many of us are so busy that we often shortchange our personal lives, neglecting our partners as well as our own needs and desires.

Lifestyle Options

Today, more than ever, there are many diverse ways of being in a relationship:

- Marriage
- Celibacy
- Celibate marriage
- Marriage without living together
- Living together without marriage
- Monogamous relationship without marriage
- Serial monogamy (being married or in a committed relationship multiple times)
- Being single but sexually active
- Homosexual relationship
- Polygamous marriage

ALERT

The divorce rate in the United States has grown steadily to 50 percent in the last several decades. There are now more second, third, and fourth marriages, and they have less of a stigma attached to them than in the past.

Westerners in particular are becoming more tolerant of diverse partnership models as the population grows and we see daily news about different groups that struggle with freedom of choice. Though some religions struggle with questions of the acceptance of nontraditional relationships, changes are occurring even in that arena.

More Information and Education

Perhaps one of the biggest changes in our modern approach to sex is the wealth of information, education, and discussion that is accessible and available. People today are much better informed about things like sexual techniques, sexual health, impotence and libido problems, and so on. And anything we don't know, we can probably easily find out. Young people today also tend to be much better informed about sex. Most kids today have at least a basic knowledge about how to protect themselves from pregnancy and STDs.

Symbols of Sex and Regeneration

Ancient men had many symbols for sex, regeneration, family, and love. Artwork dating back as long as 35,000 years depicts the importance of sex, procreation, and love in our lives, and those same themes are still prevalent in modern art. Sex has been recognized as the force that controls the universe and programs our lives, both biologically and emotionally.

The downward pointing triangle, with a small vertical slit at the bottom point, has been used as a symbol of the vulva and the female genitals since the beginning of human time. Its triangular symbol has been seen in cave drawings and carvings throughout the world. It was the first written word symbol for "female" used by the Sumerians around 3500 B.C. The phallus has been worshiped for thousands of years as the symbol of all that is male. From ancient stone megaliths, cave drawings, and objects fashioned as sex aids, the phallus symbol remains alive and well today. One need only look at our modern skyscrapers, missiles, and monuments to see how pervasive the phallus is.

Eyes: Windows to the Soul

It may be said that the eyes are a sexual symbol as well. Indeed, they are love's powerful allies. Ancient philosophies see the open eye as a metaphor for an open life and an open heart. It is said that the eyes are the seat of the soul and the gateway to the heart. Intimacy, or the act of showing one's self to another, has a direct path through the eyes.

What the Eyes Tell Us

Eyes tell truths that the tongue won't. Eighty percent of the personal energy you put out to others comes through your eyes. Humans avert their eyes when they aren't quite telling the truth or they feel uncomfortable. When people are embarrassed they tend to look away.

You can be coy with your eyes, inviting another in by looking and then looking away and then looking back. You can inflict pain and suffering with your eyes. You can hold another's gaze in a kind of game to see who will look away first. If you need alone time, you might avert your eyes, giving yourself a sense of privacy.

Pay Attention to Your Eyes

To gain a more conscious awareness of how you use your eyes, pay attention to how you use them for the next few days. Notice if you aren't willing to meet someone else's glances. Notice when you do and how it makes you feel. Try giving a person you are having a conversation with your full attention with very open, attentive eyes. See if they become more comfortable and relaxed with you.

Keep the Lights On, Baby

To enhance your intimacy and connection with your partner, keep the lights on while you make love. The lights should be soft but bright enough for the two of you to see each other well. Lie facing each other and simply let your eyes gaze at each other for five minutes. You can also try this exercise while sitting up.

FACT

The Italian anatomist Falloppio invented condoms in the sixteenth century as a way to prevent contracting syphilis. It was only later that condoms came to be used intentionally for the prevention of pregnancy. It is generally believed that condoms were first used for contraceptive purposes somewhere around the 1700s. Early condoms were made from animal skin, and would often be re-used after being washed.

This may be difficult for you, but stay with it and practice it often. Take it into your lovemaking. See the beauty in the person you are with. Very soon you will be wondering how you ever made love without having your eyes open.

Let Your Eyes Speak the Emotions

Play some eye-flirting games with your partner or with someone with whom you feel safe. You can consciously set up a game by challenging each other to display certain emotions. Ask your partner to use her or his eyes to express the different qualities of the emotions associated with rapture, longing, neediness, coyness, and devotion. Then try it yourself. Use some of these expressions in your lovemaking.

Drink in the Feelings Expressed

Receiving information with the eyes is just as important as giving information with the eyes. Keep your eyes soft and receptive. There's no need to react, raise your eyebrows, or frown. Just be. Let your partner in. Take a deep breath and relax. Develop the capacity to soften to an even deeper level.

The Myth of Eros and Psyche

The Greek myth of Eros and Psyche demonstrates the deep connection between love, sexuality, and the soul. It can serve as a source of inspiration for us even today, because it teaches the importance of intimacy and trust.

According to Greek mythology, Eros was the son of Aphrodite, the goddess of sensual love. Psyche was the youngest of three daughters and her beauty was said to rival Aphrodite's. Because of this, Aphrodite became jealous and asked Eros to have Psyche married to a monster that would devour her. But one of Eros's own arrows pricked him and he fell in love with Psyche.

Eros put her in a beautiful garden and castle and came to her only at night. He told Psyche that she was forbidden to look upon him or he would leave her forever. Eventually, Psyche disobeyed and looked at Eros, so he left her. But by this time, Psyche was pregnant. Eventually, Psyche went to Eros's mother, Aphrodite, the goddess who hated her beauty and thought she was dead. (How often does a mother think that the woman her son has chosen isn't good enough for him?)

Aphrodite gave Psyche four tasks. Though she tried her best, the tasks were so hard that each time Psyche had no choice but to give up. But nature always came to her aid in some way, helping her complete the tasks.

On the fourth and last task, Psyche fell to the ground as if dead, and Eros finally woke from his stupor and saved her by going to Zeus. Zeus helped in a way that did not interfere with his daughter, Aphrodite—he made Psyche (the Soul) immortal, and both she and Eros took their places among the gods. They experienced loss, broken trust, and separation from parents, and they grew up. They found deep, trusting, and compassionate true love, yet they had to go through a "trial by fire" to get there.

The moral of the story is that if these two seemingly cursed lovers can conquer the heavens and immortal foes to be together and enjoy love, surely there's hope for the rest of us!

Stand by Your Man (or Woman)!

The challenge today is to get through the hard times, to make it through your own personal trial by fire. It's very easy to simply give up and walk away from a relationship. The high divorce rates attest to the fact that many people choose to just cut their losses when things start going south. With so many fish in the sea and so many easy ways to meet people, there is always another woman, another man, or another relationship to move on to if this one just doesn't seem to be working.

ESSENTIAL

If you are in a loving relationship and you love sex, it's because you feel that you are getting what you want from it—deep, conscious intimacy. If you are addicted to sex, just for the physical part, you are probably afraid of intimacy.

But remember the old adage about the grass always seeming greener. No relationship is perfect. Even the best love affairs will occasionally hit a rough patch. The same struggles, drama, complaints, and problems will come up eventually. True, life is too short to waste time on a relationship that has run its course, and nobody benefits from staying together if both of you are miserable. But if you have genuine feelings for each other and are simply feeling like things have gotten a bit stale, there is plenty of hope—and this book can help bring that spark back to your relationship.

CHAPTER 3

The Body Beautiful

Ancient cultures, which held a positive view of sexuality, believed that the body is a temple. You receive your body to care for in this life. If you don't take good care of it, who will? You are at your best when you are healthy, happy, and balanced. And, of course, having a healthy body leads to great sex! In fact, aerobic fitness has been found to be one of the factors that contribute positively to both a man's and a woman's sexual experience.

Body Image in Our Culture

Let's face it, it's not easy to feel confident about your body nowadays. We're constantly bombarded with images of models and actors that have been surgically improved and plumped, plucked, injected, and enhanced to the fullest extent that modern medicine and technology can allow. And as if that's not enough, images of those models are then further enhanced using digital imaging software. Even the models themselves find it a daunting task to try and live up to their own unrealistic photos. Several supermodels have even come out and admitted to being Photoshopped in their covers, further acknowledging that in real life they have (gasp!) cellulite and other problems just like the rest of us.

ALERT

Self-consciousness and self-doubts get in the way of full sexual expression. They can occupy your mind and keep you from focusing your attention on the physical sensations that bring you pleasure. Yet many people lose themselves, agonizing over whether they're "good enough" or "pretty enough." Don't fall into this trap!

Be Realistic

It's important that you adjust your expectations for others and yourself, or you'll be inevitably disappointed when nobody can meet your impossible standards. Also, don't assume your partner expects perfection. This can be especially problematic for women, who often feel they pale in comparison to the buxom, Botox-enhanced centerfold models their men seem to drool over. In fact, many men say they'd find that overly enhanced type of women to be a turnoff in real life. Odds are, the main turn-on is that the women seem comfortable with their bodies and sexually open and adventurous.

Conquer Your Old Baggage

Unlearning the negative attitudes you inherited about bodily pleasure as a child may take time. You probably weren't encouraged to learn about your body and what brings you pleasure. When you touched yourself, an adult would move your hand away from down there.

If you received more painful negative reinforcement, you may carry guilt and shame regarding your sexual feelings, desires, and actions. Your body may carry the physical memories of those hurts just as your emotions do. It's important to understand that the hurts and injustices you may have experienced in your early years can hold you back from being a fully expressed sexual and sensual being.

Learn to Love Your Body

Pay close attention: it's important that you learn to love (or at least really like) your body. This will greatly improve your chances of having a good sex life, but it will also have a positive impact on every other part of your life. When people love their bodies, they tend to eat right, exercise, and stay healthy without worrying about the details. But getting to that place of acceptance and love so that you can nurture your body temple may be a challenge for you. Your family history, the stresses of modern life, and perfectionist ideals you hold may stop you from full acceptance. Once you become aware of your unfriendly attitudes toward your body and understand how you learned them, you can begin the journey to greater self-love.

You can start to change your negative attitudes by learning to love your body right now. If you do, you won't have to look back forty years from now and say, "Why didn't I just love myself the way I was?" Start now.

Be Open to Improvement

You can love your body while still recognizing that there's room for improvement. If you don't look or feel as good as you'd like, consider healthy ways you can make positive changes. Look for physical activities you enjoy—they will help you get in better shape, improve your mental state, and boost your self-confidence. Even better, look for activities that you and your partner can do together—allowing you both to get healthier while spending quality time together.

Begin by noticing how often you worry about what your lover might be thinking of your physical features, whether it's breasts, hips, or tummy (if you're a woman), or penis, muscles, or hair (if you're a man). Notice how you talk trash to yourself. Now start talking back. Tell yourself what you appreciate about your body. When you appreciate the gifts you have been given, you can begin the journey toward learning to love and honor your temple—just as it is.

Body Image Exercise

When you recognize that it is only you who hold yourself back, you can recover your power and discover your freedom. If you decide that as an adult you do not agree with some of the things you were taught as a child, you can make the decision to reclaim your vitality and your capacity for bodily pleasure. Here is a simple exercise that will be useful in all areas of your life:

1. Create an image in your mind of a situation or time when you felt really good about yourself. You feel empowered, smart, and capable.
2. Close your eyes and breathe deeply into your belly for a few minutes while you hold on to that feeling. Really feel it and breathe it in.
3. Now, imagine that you are feeling that way about your body: It is strong; it is healthy; and it is beautiful. Drink in that feeling and bathe yourself in it for a few minutes.

You'll find training for increasing the pleasure you feel in your many erogenous zones in an upcoming chapter, but for now, know that this little exercise will vastly improve your sex life. Practice loving yourself!

Take Care of Yourself

When you view your body as a temple, you honor and hold it sacred. When you feel sacred and honored, you feel good about yourself. And when you feel good, you're more able to experience your fullest sexual pleasure.

Today we live in ever-increasing "busy-ness." The thing we all want more of is time, and the demands on your time are much different than they were even in your parents' generation. In general, commutes are longer, school events are more common, and two-income households are the norm rather than the exception. Adults will often put themselves last on a list of the things that must be done in a day. There are the children and the jobs, dinner, offices, laundry, and so much more—the list goes on and on. But who's taking care of the caretaker? You must take care of yourself, or you won't be able to care for anyone else. As the caretaker, you are relied upon, so you must take care of yourself.

Here's a hint about time: It all comes down to priorities. There is time for the things you really value when you schedule them in. You put meetings, project dates, social events, work, and your favorite TV show on your calendar, so why not schedule time for a long, sensual bath? Value yourself as you value these other things. Plan time for yourself and put it on your schedule. Soon it will get to be a habit.

ESSENTIAL

Take a long bath. Put on music. Take a glass of sparkling apple cider in with you. Put a few drops of an essential oil in the tub. Pour in some bubble bath. Sprinkle in a few fresh rose petals from the garden. Any one of these things is so simple and yet will relax you and make you feel special.

Do some stretching or yoga. Give your feet a little attention. After all, they are your foundation. Give them a pedicure or massage them. Find something for yourself that is a treat and make time for it. Everyone in your life will be happier you did.

Try Another Body Image Exercise

Find an hour to yourself, a time when you'll have quiet and peace. Take a shower or a bath. Wash yourself lovingly and really feel your skin on your thighs, your chest, your buttocks, and your face. Let your fingertips move slowly and lightly over your skin. Your fingers should be enjoying the touch of your own body. Towel-dry and put on a soft robe.

Go into the room that has the largest mirror in your home and do the following:

1. Gaze softly into the reflection of your eyes for a few moments. (This may seem difficult or awkward, but don't be afraid to try it.)
2. Smile softly at yourself. Breathe deeply.
3. Separate the front of your robe and look at your body, slowly, with focus and attention. Notice all of the parts that you like. Why do you like each part? Has a lover said that he likes that part?
4. Take an inventory of the places and parts that you like and the reasons you like them. Now, what parts are you not happy with? Why? What is it about those parts and places that you don't like? Can you identify whether these parts really don't satisfy you, or whether your judgment has been affected by cultural stereotypes of how you're supposed to look?
5. If you have any complaints about your body, say them out loud. Say them again, for as many times as it takes for you to understand that that is all they are—complaints. We start sounding a little ridiculous to ourselves when we repeat a complaint again and again. Do this now and do it up big time: complain, complain, and complain!

When you've finished, ask yourself how you feel. Simply expressing a feeling can often help it dissolve or change. Can you gaze upon your body with a little more acceptance and love? Spend just a final moment gazing in the mirror again. Relax, smile, and thank yourself for the new level of understanding you have achieved.

The Capacity for Pleasure

The truth is that you have the same working parts that everyone else has, and that is all it takes for great sex. One culture will love big bottoms, another will love small breasts, and yet another will prefer hairless men. It doesn't matter what happens to be in vogue in your present time and place. You've got what you've got and your friend has what she has.

When you realize this, you'll be free to be in your body and experience what it is capable of. When you consider that your brain is your biggest erogenous zone, you start to think about how little you might actually be feeling, and you can begin using your body to its fullest pleasure capacity. When you get past focusing on your shortcomings, then you can begin to have access to your full pleasure.

Erotic Presence

Some people need help bringing out their erotic presence, the way you radiate your erotic nature. This is not to say that you must become alluring, coy, and seductive, but rather that you become aware of your capacity for a natural eroticism. Grace, energy, and confidence allude to an erotic nature. Take the opportunity to notice what your style is and how you might develop it.

If you go dancing, try upping the ante a little. Don't worry about technique; consciously throw yourself more fully into the steps and the swing. Be the dance. Let the energy flow through you.

If you feel self-conscious about erotic presence, try dancing at home just for yourself. Choose a time and place where you have privacy. For both men and women, you might want to dress in a sarong or something a bit sexy. Find a scarf or a hat or a feathery boa you can wave around. Put on music with a good rhythm and start to move. You can dance in front of a mirror if you'd like.

Do a Body Wave

Stop censoring your movement—just let yourself go. Try a new move. Wave your arms around. Keep it light. Loosen your pelvis with some body waves. To do these, stand with your feet a little apart and bend your knees. Relax. As you begin the movement, stick your bottom out and then gently swing your hips forward. When you feel comfortable with this, begin to let your upper body move to the wave. Your spine will become looser and the wave will move up to your neck and head. Do this slowly and begin to smooth out the movements as you repeat it. Let your head go and include the natural action of your arms. Go with the flow.

ESSENTIAL

Add a little lingerie to your lovemaking. Women can try wearing a demibra or a push-up bra, especially when they are on top. Men can keep their silk boxers or a muscle shirt on while making love. Not showing everything or hinting at what's beneath can be just as erotic as making love in the buff.

This is an excellent way to warm up for lovemaking. You may even get to the place of being able to dance for your lover. Pretend you are a temple dancer. What better erotic foreplay could you imagine?

With a little practice it will become easier for you to let yourself go. You'll begin to notice other areas in your life where you can apply this same idea. The big shift will be apparent in your lovemaking, but a sense of erotic presence will energize your whole life. Find opportunities to be graceful and confident. Notice how you might add a bit of spice to that moment—especially if your partner is around to reap the benefits.

Erogenous Zones

Your whole body is one big erogenous zone. Touch applied to your hair follicles and nerves on the skin travels to the brain and is translated to erotic, sensual feelings of pleasure. But some areas are more sensitive than others, so your body's erogenous zone can generally be divided into three different types:

1. **Primary (first-degree) erogenous zone.** These include the mucous membrane tissues that comprise the lips, genitals, and nipples. These areas include the anus, penis, vaginal lips, and inside the outer third of the vagina. They are rich in nerves and the nerve endings are very close to the surface of the skin. These areas are very responsive to touch.

2. **Secondary (second-degree) erogenous zone.** Parts that have a sparse amount of hair and are often found in the regions next to the third-degree areas. These parts are not as sensitive as the primary erogenous zone, but are more sensitive than the areas covered by hair.

3. **Tertiary (third-degree) erogenous zone.** The areas of the skin that are covered with hair—your arms, legs, parts of the chest, and so forth. These areas have fewer and more dispersed nerve endings, so they are the least erogenous. Nevertheless, the hair follicles' ends, down under the skin, help stimulate the nerve endings that are buried near them.

ESSENTIAL

The word erogenous comes to us from the Greeks. *Ero* comes from Eros, the name of the Greek god of erotic love, and *genous* is a suffix that means producing or generating. Erogenous zones are areas that generate erotic love.

Humans need touch from the time they are born to become healthy individuals. Our skin and nerves grow in their ability to feel more fully as we develop. This process can be expanded your whole life long. You will always have the ability to increase your capacity to feel the pleasure of touch.

Mutual Enjoyment: A Key to Great Touch

A key ingredient to great touch is this rule: The hand that gives the touch should feel just as good (or better) than the body part receiving the touch. In other words, the giver should be in pleasure along with the receiver. Think about this—it's quite a concept. The next time you give pleasurable touch to a person, think about your fingertips. Are they enjoying themselves? How could they be enjoying this experience even more?

When you start paying attention, you will find that you can really enjoy being the giver. You'll find new ways to touch that will open up the experience for both of you. This simple practice will transform sensual touch for you *and* your partner. It even works when the giver and the receiver is the same person. Try it in a fun way; be light and playful.

Don't Overlook the Less Obvious Zones

One common mistake people make is focusing on a few obvious parts of the body, ignoring many other perfectly good potential hotspots. Explore your partner's (and your own) body, giving every nook and cranny a chance to be the Erogenous Zone of the Day. You just might find a few surprises. Remember, erogenous zones are an individual thing. What might not do anything for one person will drive another person up the wall.

The Pleasure of Touch

Here is a fun exercise for increasing erotic, physical pleasure through touch. You can do this alone or with a partner as an experiential evening of erotic play. If you do it with a partner, it will involve direct sexual activity. Make sure you lovingly communicate what is and isn't working for you. If you are practicing solo, you can self-pleasure your genitals with one hand and stimulate other erogenous zones with the other hand.

The training idea behind this practice is to make new or deeper neural connections between the excitement you feel in your genital area and other areas of your body. For instance, let's take a basic example. Women, let's connect the pleasure you feel in your clitoris with your nipples. You or your partner would stimulate your clitoris to the point of arousal and then begin to simultaneously stimulate your nipples in whatever way you like. This could be orally or with either of you using your fingers and hands.

Men, you would be stimulating your penis and your nipples. If you are doing it with your lover, have your partner stimulate your penis and you can arouse your nipples or any area of your choice. Remember to breathe fully into your belly. Keep the stimulation up. Take it to the arousal point and then some. Breathe in the pleasurable energy.

Next, continue the genital stimulation but switch to another erogenous zone. Connect each new area with the direct genital excitement you are feeling. Some areas will work better than others, but remember that every inch of your skin is covered in nerve endings that can learn to experience more pleasure. Even the areas between your fingers and toes are exquisitely tender and sensitive when touched lightly and playfully.

More Erogenous Areas

Here are a few other erogenous areas you may concentrate on as you perform this exercise:

- Breasts and underarms
- Toes and feet
- Buttocks and anus
- Inner and outer thighs
- Neck area, ears, and face

- Love handles and sides of the torso
- Back of the knees and inside the elbows
- Fingers and wrists

ALERT

Let your imagination run wild, but be respectful of your partner and her likes or dislikes. Remember to ask permission to touch an area you think might be risky or extra-sensitive. Speak up if something feels less than pleasurable—or if something feels so good you want more of it.

By working on your secondary and tertiary erogenous zones, you are training your body to feel much more. After some practice, it is even conceivable to reach orgasm just by having your nipples sucked. The possibilities are endless!

When the breath is connected to this practice, it too can be used as the vehicle to orgasm. Eventually, it may even be possible for you to breathe the way you did during this exercise and reach orgasm without physical contact. This is not far-fetched and is, in fact, a common practice in tantra. Can you imagine how beneficial this will be in helping you achieve an orgasm *with* genital stimulation?

CHAPTER 4

Intimacy as a Spiritual Voyage

The word intimacy comes from the Latin *intimatus*, meaning to make something known to someone else. When you make yourself known to someone else, you are contributing to deeper intimacy. Intimacy isn't about doing things and going places together as much as it's about being together. Close experiences, relying on each other, talking, and sharing hurts and frustrations—that's intimacy. Revealing yourself (both literally and figuratively) can strengthen your sexual and romantic bond. An intimate sexual relationship is both a journey to know your partner and a journey to know yourself.

Dealing with Fears of Intimacy

Everyone has one or two favorite fears. For some people one is rejection. For others, it's abandonment or betrayal. Then there's the fear of being misunderstood or not being heard, and, of course, the old standby, being smothered or controlled. These fears originate in childhood, but even when we become adults, fears have a way of finding their way into the bedroom.

FACT

An intimate sexual relationship can provide a safe place to uncover and own up to your fears. While this might not sound like much fun, it is very valuable. When you can admit and speak about your fears to your partner, this is a big first step toward healing whatever early wounding led to the fear in the first place.

Recognize Your Fear

Here is an example: When Lila was a little girl, her mother ignored her when she cried loudly for what she wanted. As a result, Lila came to the unfortunate conclusion that it wasn't safe to ask for what she wanted. Now, in bed with Steve, she is hoping he'll stroke her head as part of their foreplay. But she can't force herself to ask, because she is afraid he will just ignore her. Instead, she attempts to override her desire and just enjoy the feeling of Steve's hands on other parts of her body.

The only trouble is, Lila isn't really able to push her real desire out of her thoughts and cannot be fully present to enjoy Steve's touch. She's in her head, worrying about what to do, rather than in her body, enjoying this present moment with her lover. When you have a feeling that you try to push away, it usually won't go. This is especially true if the feeling is related to a childhood-based fear that needs to be addressed and healed.

Conquer Your Fear

If you find yourself in a situation similar to Lila's, first gently remind yourself that the beliefs you learned in childhood about what is and isn't safe are not true. That was then, and this is now. When you were little and dependent, it was indeed scary if you asked for something and got ignored. As a child you were totally dependent on the adults around you for your very survival. Now you are a self-supporting adult.

If Lila asks Steve to stroke her head and he ignores her, or if he does it but not the way she really likes, she will survive. So the idea that it's not safe to ask for what you want is an old, outdated belief that she now has the opportunity to heal or outgrow. If she asks and doesn't get what she wants, at least her asking gets her back into the present time with herself and her lover.

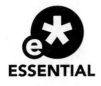

ESSENTIAL

The healing comes not so much from asking and getting, but from asking and finding out that just the act of asking is an act of affirming yourself. Becoming self-validating or self-affirming is what adults do. Waiting for someone else to make you happy is what children do.

If you decide to take the risk and ask for what you want, it's often a good idea to mention that you are feeling some fear associated with asking—that you are feeling tentative and vulnerable due to old fears in your mind. Letting your partner know that your fears are about you and not him can help him not to take your feelings personally.

Voice Your Concerns

Here is how an intimate request like this might go: "I'm feeling very close to you, and I'm also feeling that I want to ask you to touch me in a particular way . . . but I'm afraid to ask. I know this fear is something very old, something I've always had, long before you and I met. So what I want is for you to stroke my head just like you were doing last night while we were watching TV. It always feels so special when you do that for me."

Mentioning your fear out loud also helps you accept yourself just as you are. And it helps you take your fear less seriously and get over it. After expressing a feeling, the feeling usually changes. Funny how that works!

Past Problems That Can Interfere with Intimacy

The sad fact is, it's tough to let go of certain remnants of past relationships. We all carry old baggage and perhaps a few scars from relationships gone bad. It's important to address this history—and the role it may play in your current relationships—if you want to move on and enjoy a healthy and satisfying relationship with your current partner.

Old Baggage That Can Haunt You

Here are some types of past relationships (and relationship problems) that can hinder your ability to be truly intimate with your current partner:

- **Parental issues.** If you've had problematic parental relationships, this can be a lifelong obstacle to happy relationships if you don't learn to deal with it. Common problems include parental abandonment or absence, an abusive parent, and a parent who didn't show emotion or affection. On the opposite end of the spectrum is the overly affection or too-attached parent who may have trouble cutting the cord, thus making it difficult for you to fully devote yourself to a romantic relationship.
- **Abusive partners.** If a past partner was abusive in any way—physically, mentally or verbally—it may be very tough for you to trust another partner and let your guard down. You need to recognize that the abuser was to blame for her actions, and you weren't responsible for her behavior. You also can't assume your current partner will treat you the same way.
- **Relationships lacking passion or affection.** If you had a previous relationship that lacked a spark, you may have gotten accustomed to that status quo, so you might need to make an extra effort to rekindle that Romeo or sex kitten that is buried inside you but is dying to be set free.

ALERT

If negative experiences and attitudes from previous relationships are weighing you down, it might be a good idea to seek a counselor or therapist who can help you deal with those issues so you can give your current or future relationship the best possible chance to succeed.

The Role of Emotions

If you just want to spice up your sex life, you may wonder why so much of this material deals with emotions. That's easy: It's nearly impossible to separate the mind and body when it comes to having a terrific, satisfying sexual encounter. Okay, a quickie or one-night-stand might not require a deep, intimate bond (although you might be surprised at how much emotions can come into play, even in supposedly casual encounters). But for any type of lasting or serious relationship, emotions play a big role in fulfilling and enjoyable lovemaking.

If you and your partner feel a mutual respect, affection, and trust for each other, you are much more likely to surrender your hearts, souls, and bodies completely to each other. You are also much more willing to consider new or daring sexual experiences and techniques.

Even seemingly negative emotions can spark hot lovemaking with someone who you care deeply about. How many times have you enjoyed raw, animalistic sex immediately after a heated argument? Or had some slow, tender make-up sex once you've settled your dispute?

Sexual Vulnerability

If you want to have great sex and experience intimacy, a willingness to be sexually vulnerable is a must. Most people protect themselves when they are around other people. This is true even in sex. We tend to be wary of others hurting us, so we keep a layer of protection around our hearts just in case. Then, if a partner does something that we associate with rejection, criticism, or any of our other favorite fears, we say, "I knew it! I knew this would happen! It's a good thing I didn't let myself get completely vulnerable—because then, I'd be even more hurt."

Opening up to your partner is an act of great trust. It is the most important thing you can do for yourself if you want to heal your old wounds and realize that you can trust yourself to deal with whatever happens to you.

Being openly vulnerable can also help you see that the pain another person's behavior triggers in you tells you that you still need to heal in yourself. Pain is not necessarily bad; it can reveal to you the areas in your unconscious belief structure that need to be updated. It shows you where you need to focus in your journey toward wholeness.

What are your areas of potential vulnerability with respect to sex and lovemaking? For many people, the idea of asking for what they want is the big one. You heard about one way of dealing with this fear in the example of Lila and Steve. Another way is to simply ask for what you want while feeling your fear, but not explicitly speaking about it. Experiment with both approaches. Sometimes one way will be more real for you, and at other times the other way will feel better.

Let Go of Your Fears and Inhibition

There are other ways of being sexually vulnerable. Just allowing your partner to see exactly what you are thinking and feeling is a wonderful gift—to both of you. Some people are afraid of not looking good when they are in the heat of passion. If you have this fear, talk to your partner about it. It is very likely you will be reassured to know that most people feel honored to be trusted with that level of vulnerability from someone they love.

Other ways to practice being open and vulnerable are:

- Look into each other's eyes while in the heat of passion.
- Tell your partner exactly how something that she is doing feels.
- Let your partner know when you are feeling unsatisfied or when you are in a state of longing for more closeness (without blaming your partner for your feeling).
- Ask your partner for feedback about what you are doing to pleasure her (with an attitude of sincerely wanting to please).

Practice Enhancing Intimacy

This might surprise you, but intimacy doesn't always come easily, even with someone you love. But you can create intimacy between you and your partner through effort and practice. There are several exercises that will help you enhance intimacy in your relationship and build on your self-knowledge.

Creating Safe, Sacred Space

It's tough to truly relax and open yourself up to another person if you are tense or uncomfortable in your environment. This is especially important with your romantic relationships. You and your partner should have your own special love nest where you can enjoy each other's company without distractions or annoyances. That's why you need to create your sensual, sacred space. This is where you go to enjoy sensual lovemaking or talk about matters of importance. To sanctify this space, you might light a candle, burn some incense, or smudge by burning herbs. Whenever you enter this space, even if there is disharmony in the air, you enter it with an attitude of openness to *what is*—willing to speak about and hear whatever is ready to be revealed.

Spend Quality Time in Your Space

Your sacred space isn't doing any good if your hardly use it. Even if your schedules are very busy, make it a point to spend some time alone together doing something fun in your sacred space. Ideally, this would mean leisurely lovemaking sessions, but it could also include quickies, massages, adult games, watching romantic/erotic movies, or whatever else you two enjoy doing together.

Overcoming Differences

The intimate journey of two people toward wholeness will inevitably involve differences and conflict about these differences. Communicating openly about these differences can feel scary, and that's normal. But open communication can also lead to an actual expansion of each individual's sense of the self, resulting in a deeper sense of unity, not only with each other, but with all of life as well. To illustrate how this happens, here is a true story of a couple conflicted about the issue of whether to continue their monogamous relationship or to switch to a more open lifestyle.

Paula is fifty. Paul is forty-six. They have been married for ten years; this is the second marriage for both. When they first got together, they agreed to be monogamous, but now things have changed. Paul believes he has only a few good years left in terms of his sexual vitality. He has had four sexual partners in his life, and he's feeling a need to experiment with other lovers.

He also has the idea that being monogamous is killing his passion and his sense of vitality as a man. He sincerely believes that it is dishonest for him to pretend to be satisfied with just one sex partner. He loves Paula and enjoys what the two of them have together, but he keeps noticing his sexual attention being drawn toward other women.

Paula is beside herself with grief and anger. She wants to stay monogamous. She believes that sex is a sacred act, and she has not had any desire to be with other sex partners.

ESSENTIAL

If you can stay in the impasse long enough, allowing the difference to exist rather than rushing prematurely to a resolution, you will be changed by the experience. This change is not predictable. It doesn't take the form of giving in or compromising but rather of expanding yourself.

As a result, the couple is at an impasse. Paul feels strongly that he cannot be true to himself and stay monogamous. He also feels genuine empathy for Paula. It hurts him to see her in pain. Paula imagines that if Paul has sex with other women, she will not be able to be as open and vulnerable with him. She trusts what Paul says about himself—that he feels dishonest pretending to want to be monogamous. She wants Paul to have what he wants, and, at the same time, she thinks she'd be untrue to herself staying in a nonmonogamous relationship.

What Would You Do?

If you were Paul or Paula, can you imagine how you might experience such a predicament? Can you imagine feeling two contradictory things at once: the wish to have what you want alongside the wish for your partner to have what she wants? This is often what it feels like to hold differences. It's like being in an unresolved predicament without knowing if there will be a resolution.

A Good Resolution

In Paul and Paula's case, they stayed with their pain and uncertainty for about six months. Then they both stated that they felt a sense of ego transcendence. Paul discovered that his need for other lovers was actually connected to some unresolved anger at both Paula and at his mother. After he was able to express his anger to both of them and to get over it, here's what Paul had to say about the experience: "What I thought I needed for my survival doesn't seem so crucial now." Paula also got a deeper look at herself after staying with her pain. She remembered a time early in the marriage when Paul broke one of his agreements with her—an agreement that had to do with money, not sex. After she cleared this up with Paul, by expressing her resentment, she then saw that breaking agreements had been a trigger for her all her life. She did some crying and grieving for some of the disappointments she had felt as a child. Afterward, she was finally free enough of old baggage to say truthfully, "I feel a lot safer, like my security doesn't depend on other people, like I'll be okay if the relationship ends, even though I still very much want to be with Paul."

Outcomes like this often feel magical or unbelievable to the people involved—when they consider where they were before they got unstuck. For so many, just staying in the impasse, holding their differences for a period of time, produces an inner expansion or transformation that enables them to experience a deeper level of what's real for each of them.

Practice Holding Your Differences

To help you experience holding differences, pick an unresolved conflict between you and your partner. Sit facing each other. Let's say one partner opens the dialogue by sharing something she resents about the other partner. She begins by using the sentence structure, "I resent you for . . . " and then sharing bodily sensations, self-talk, or anything else related to the resentment. Her partner actively listens, mirroring back what he has just heard.

What is active listening?
It's a communication practice that helps you stay present to what your partner is saying without getting defensive. It also lets your partner know that you are attempting to hear her accurately.

Then, when the woman says she is satisfied with how her partner listened to her, he shares what he is experiencing right in the moment. He does not debate the content of her message. His experience can be whatever he feels, thinks, or says to himself after hearing what his partner said. The woman actively listens and then shares her present experience. They keep going back and forth like this for five to ten minutes.

A Sample Conversation

Here's an example of how you could conduct your conversation:

- **Dan:** I resent you for not initiating sex with me more often. You've only approached me three times in the past six months. I feel like I am not a priority in your life.
- **Dora:** You resent me for not initiating sex. You feel like you're not a priority in my life. Is that what you said? [Dan nods.] Okay. I resent you for saying I never initiate sex.
- **Dan:** You resent me for saying you never initiate sex. Did I hear you correctly? [Dora nods.] And I resent you for saying the word "never." I didn't say you never initiate. I said you have done it three times in the last six months.
- **Dora:** You're saying you resent me for saying "never," and that what you really said was I only initiated three times in the last six months. Did I get it? [Dan nods.] And I'm feeling sad. I'm saying to myself that I'm not so good at initiating even though I'd like to. I'm unsure of myself in the arena that you're so good in.
- **Dan:** You're feeling sad and you're thinking that you don't have confidence in your ability to initiate sex. Is that right? [Dora nods.] And right now I'm feeling softer toward you.

- **Dora:** You say you're feeling softer toward me. Yes? [Dan nods.] I'm feeling a little bit softer and more relaxed now, too.

In this example, Dan and Dora started out resenting each other and ended up feeling softer toward each other. Things don't always happen this way, but they often do. This sort of change is most likely to happen when the two people stay present to what the other has just said and share their here-and-now response. Paying careful attention to your own experience and to each other allows you to experience feelings more fully so that they can be released. It also teaches you both the art of holding differences.

Overcoming Long-Term Conflict

If you and your partner have a long history of conflict, it would be a good idea to try this exercise with another person or pair observing. Having a witness or witnesses helps you stay with the exercise, which can be very difficult. Couples are accustomed to bypassing their present experience and going immediately into their interpretations, generalizations, stereotypes, knee-jerk reactions, and self-protective judgments about each other. It's highly unusual for people to simply share their present experiences.

ESSENTIAL

If the pain or tension of holding differences becomes too great, it's okay to agree to set the subject aside for several days or even weeks. Agree to revisit the issue and agree on a time in the future. When that time comes, make sure you do come back to the discussion, even if it is uncomfortable.

Dan and Dora's conversation took place between a real person and another real person instead of between one's interpretation and the other's interpretation. The latter would look more like this: "You don't care about my needs. I've told you a hundred times what I want." (This is an interpretation followed by a generalization. He can't really know what she does or does not care about.) "Well, you don't care about my needs either! You never treat me with respect." (Another interpretation and another generalization.) Does this sound familiar?

If you've been in a relationship for any length of time, it probably does! Mates who have been together for a while tend to camouflage the really painful unfinished situations by making interpretations, generalizations, comparisons, and assessments. They apparently hope that this sort of more distant, less intimate language will keep them a safe distance from the pain.

Holding differences trains you to tolerate more intensity of feeling, whether it is painful or pleasurable. As a practice, it helps you stay with the discomfort and fully experience the moment, until you achieve clarity. It also helps partners discover what is real for each other, instead of getting caught up defending their interpretations and stereotypes. Using active listening with the intent of staying in your experience is a very effective tool for helping you to stick to *what is*, rather than escaping into explanations or defensiveness.

A Connection with Your Partner

As you embark on your voyage toward greater intimacy and mutual awareness, you can practice positions of nurturing that will help you to restore and harmonize your energies after a fight or disagreement. And if you still don't feel comfortable doing these with your partner, practice on your own, in front of a mirror.

Eye Gazing

Choose a quiet place. Sit in a comfortable position, with you and your partner facing each other. Preferably, you are on cushions on the floor, sitting cross-legged and face-to-face, as close to each other as possible. You may sit on chairs with a straight back so you sit up straight. Relax and breathe into your belly.

Look at your partner. Your eyes should be soft and inviting. You don't have to smile or look fascinated—just relax, breathe, and allow yourself to open up to the moment. Stay together in this way for about five minutes.

FACT

One of the benefits of eye gazing at close range and breathing to-gether is the exchange of pheromones, the sexual scents that induce arousal. They are passed through bodily secretions and the breath. When you are engaged in activities that promote pheromone release, you will develop stronger bonds.

Next, each of you should place your right hand on your partner's heart and your left hand over your partner's arm, on your own heart. The palms of your hands should be flat so that they are touching your partner and your-self completely. Breathe and eye gaze. Relax into the feeling of complete surrender. Stay present with your partner and focus your awareness on only the two of you.

Examine Your Experience

After you have tried eye gazing, think about how this exercise affected you. Here are a few questions you may want to ask yourself:

- Did I have any trouble looking into my partner's eyes? Did I only look at one and not the other?
- How did it make me feel?
- Was I comfortable or uncomfortable?
- Would I be able to sustain this exercise for five to ten minutes?

Also talk to your partner about this exercise. Share your feelings and ask how he felt about it.

Eye gazing during the act of sex is a very powerful experience. We are open and vulnerable at that time. Once you are more comfortable with doing it, see if you can look into your lover's eyes while you orgasm. This may be more difficult—you're probably conditioned to go inside, thinking you'll feel the experience more. In truth, you may actually be able to expand the orgasmic feelings more when you are fully connected to your partner through your eyes.

Heart Hold While Spooning

This is an excellent exercise to clear negative energy that can arise from everyday fights and disagreements. Lie on your side with your partner, with one of you in front of the other, like spoons in a drawer. If you are in back, place your top arm over your partner and hold your hand to her heart. If you are in front, have your partner place her hand on your heart. Relax and breathe together. Do this for at least five minutes.

After a few minutes, you can also try some slow, gentle undulating together. One of you starts and begins to rock from the hips. Cradle your partner in your arms and hold firmly. This is a good tool for getting in sync or harmonizing.

CHAPTER 5

A Woman's Body

The female sexual anatomy has been likened to a flower. Her parts are delicate, sturdy, exotic, soft, intriguing, and colorful—all at the same time. A woman's sex organs must be strong and resilient enough to bear children. Yet they are also exquisitely sensitive during the act of lovemaking. A women's private anatomical area is beautiful and unique, functional and deliberately designed. But, most importantly for lovemaking, it is filled with sensitive parts capable of feeling overwhelming ecstasy.

Woman: A Unique Being

Female sexuality is a complicated thing. The woman is the only animal who is able to conceive during a portion of every month, all year round. When the issue of sexual intercourse comes up, most heterosexual women under the age of fifty must also consider the issue of possible pregnancy. Sex is not simply an act of sharing intimacy or pleasure, since it also carries the possibility of pregnancy.

A woman's primary sexual response mechanism is her genitals, but she has many secondary and tertiary sexual parts. In fact, every inch of her body can be very responsive to touch—especially her breasts, nipples, buttocks, hips, neck, and face.

During heightened arousal, a woman's chest, vulva, and face will often change color. The sexual flush is due to increased blood flow in these areas. It's easiest to see the flushing in these spots because the skin is particularly sensitive and somewhat thinner. When pink skin turns to deep red, this can be seen as a sign of sexual readiness.

Unlike men, women's sexual parts are diminutive and somewhat hidden, especially before sexual stimulation. They're not easily found and investigated. Women are generally taught not to touch or explore themselves; often, they aren't familiar with even the most basic information about their own bodies. Statistically, the more a woman knows her own parts and explores her sexual response, the more orgasmic she will be.

Outer Genital Area

Known as the vulva, the exterior genitals are made up of the pubis, mons veneris, the labia, and the vestibule.

The *pubis* is the triangle of hair that covers the genitals. The skin of the pubis is quite sensitive and the multiple hair follicles are receptive to sensual touch. Gentle stroking, rubbing, and even light pulling have a very erotic feel when combined with sexual stimulation of the vulva and clitoris.

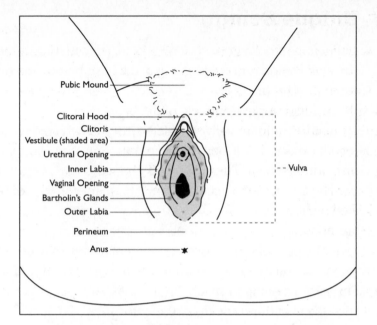

The outer area of the female genitals.

Some women and their partners like to shave the pubis area, finding this virgin look to be erotic. Keep in mind, though, that if you decide to try shaving, you may be missing the experience of the erotic feel that the hair follicles add to the sexual experience. The ancient Chinese considered thick, abundant pubic hair to be a sign of sensuality and passion.

FACT

The vulva (exterior parts) is the area of the female genitals that is exposed, or on the outside of her body. The vagina (inner parts) is the area inside her body. A woman's reproductive parts are buried even farther inside the body, beyond the vagina.

Underneath the pubis is the pubic bone, which covers the interior genitals and protects them from exterior injury. It helps support the front area of the vagina and offers the pivot point for the man to rub against during sexual intercourse. Covering the bone is the fatty tissue known as the *mons veneris*, or the *mound of Venus*. The tissue provides a cushion for the pubic bone.

The Labia

The *labia majora* and *labia minora* are the tissues that form the lips of the vulva. The *labia majora* are the larger lips that have hair on the outer side and are smooth and hairless on the inner side. These lips protect the delicate tissue of the inner lips and the rest of the vulva.

As the genitals become sexually stimulated, the labia majora will become engorged with blood and will begin to separate and open to expose the inner sanctuary of the vulva. The tissue will change color as sexual excitement mounts. The typically pink skin will turn to deeper shades of pink as it becomes filled with blood.

The labia minora are the more delicate inner lips of the vulva. Here begins the mucous membrane, smooth tissue that is hairless and pink. This tissue is soft and porous and has many more nerves than the outer tissue of the labia majora. This skin forms the inner lips that meet at the top of the vulva and form the hood over the tip of the clitoris.

The inner lips contain sweat glands and scent glands that secrete moisturizers to lubricate the vulva and pheromones to signal sexual readiness. As the genitals fill with blood, the lubrication is literally squeezed out by the pressure buildup in the tissue. The pressure can build to such a degree that the lubrication can actually flow out of the vagina, making it easier to insert the penis during lovemaking.

The Clitoris

The clitoris is actually much larger than it appears. Most of it is buried on the inside of the woman's body, so the hood and the clitoral tip are all we see. The inner part is reminiscent of a smaller penis; it is a shaft that splits into two forks, or *crura* (legs), as it goes deeper into the body. The urethral sponge, or G-spot, sits between the two crura.

The clitoris, its shaft, and the crura are composed of the same spongy material that makes up the penis. During arousal, it expands with blood and causes an erection of the clitoral tissue. The clitoris has the highest concentration of nerves of any part of the body, male or female.

Clitoral Hood and Tip

The clitoral hood is a movable fold of skin that is formed by the tissue of the labia minora where it meets at the top of the vulva. It covers the clitoral tip and the portion of the clitoris (or clitoral shaft) that is buried under the skin.

The clitoral tip is the exposed part of the clitoris. It is rich in nerve endings and is made up of spongy tissue that holds blood during sexual excitement. It can increase greatly in size during sexual stimulation and will also change color as it becomes engorged with blood. The clitoral tip is perhaps the most sensitive part of the female body.

Vestibule

The doorway to the vagina, the vestibule, is the area that is surrounded by the labia minora. It contains the opening to the urethra, the entrance to the vagina, and the glands that secrete lubrication and scent.

FACT

The Bartholin's, or vestibular, glands secrete lubrication and produce a scent that is thought to carry the pheromones of sexual excitement. These glands, which open into the vestibule of the vagina, are the source of the vagina's musky or earthy scent.

Perineum

The perineum is the area located between the anus and the opening of the vagina. It is rich in nerves and sensitive to the touch. The perineum is a place on both men and women that can be pressed or stroked for added sexual excitement.

Inner Genital Area

The vagina is the interior portion of the woman's genitals. The vagina is deeply folded and is the area the penis enters during intercourse. The tissue is highly elastic in nature and can accommodate a wide variety of penis sizes. During sexual excitement the vagina narrows at the first third and can expand and lengthen toward the back.

The vagina is typically between 3 to 4 inches deep. If a woman who has a smaller-than-average vagina is matched with a man with a larger-than-average penis (longer than 7 inches), the couple will have to get creative with positions and stimulation techniques to relax the woman, allowing her to open more fully.

Most women and men are not very familiar with the inside of the vagina. It helps to know about these parts—both for sexual enhancement and health reasons. Here are some of the main parts of the vagina.

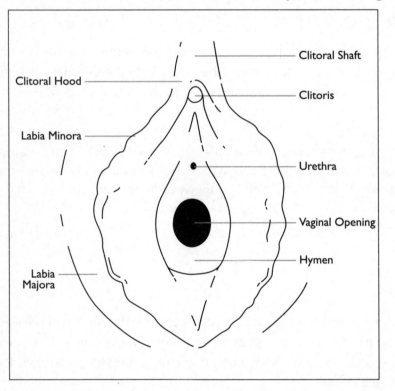

The inner female genitals, including the hymen and urethra.

The Hymen

The *hymen* is a flap of tissue that covers the entrance to the vagina, and it is present in most (but not all) virginal women. This thin membrane is broken at the time of first intercourse—or during a strenuous physical activity—and is then dissolved.

Urethra, Urethral Sponge, and G-Spot

The *urethra* is the canal, or tube, that carries urine from the bladder out of the body. It is short and ends just above the vestibule, or entrance to the vagina, below the clitoris. The urethra runs through the urethral sponge, or G-spot. It is also believed to be the delivery source for female ejaculate.

Many medical professionals still speculate on the existence of the G-spot, or G-area. Most doctors and sex educators now acknowledge that the G-spot exists. It is made up of several glands, including the female prostatic gland, blood vessels, spongy material that holds fluids, and ducts that deliver the fluids out of the body.

This area is located just inside the vaginal opening, on the top part of the vagina, directly beyond the area of rough, bumpy skin that pads the pubic bone. It is behind the pubic bone, tucked against the back side of it.

Cervix and Os

The *cervix* is the protective tip of the uterus. The *os*, or entrance to the uterus, is at its center. The cervix can be felt inside the vagina and is sometimes bumped during rough sex, causing pain.

The os typically remains very small, but changes wondrously to stretch and open up to more than 10 centimeters during childbirth. During the conception of a baby, the sperm from the father must travel through the os to get to the uterus and then on to the fallopian tubes. Menstrual blood passes out through the os and then the cervix during a woman's monthly cycle.

Reproductive Organs

A woman's reproductive parts are hidden and well protected. In addition to their reproductive role, these organs also play a vital part in hormonal distribution and regulation, thus affecting female libido and monthly cycles of fertility and responsiveness.

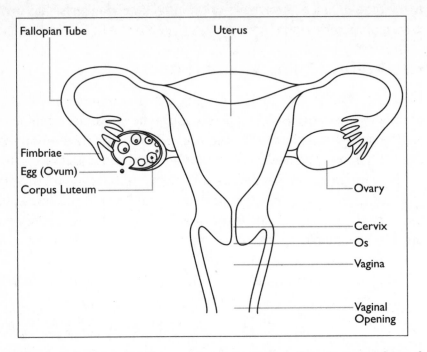

Fallopian Tube

Uterus

Fimbriae

Egg (Ovum)

Corpus Luteum

Ovary

Cervix

Os

Vagina

Vaginal Opening

The female reproductive anatomy, including the uterus and ovaries.

Uterus

The uterus is where the fertilized egg lives and develops for approximately nine months before birth. The tissue that forms the uterus is made up of powerful muscles that expand or contract according to need, with soft tissue on the inside to protect and nourish the growing fetus. The uterus is small when the woman is not pregnant—about the size of a pear—but it can stretch to considerable size when holding one or more babies.

Every month during a woman's menstrual cycle the uterus fills with blood and tissue in order to prepare for possible fertilization. If the egg is not fertilized, the blood leaves the body in the form of the woman's menstrual period. The cycle then begins again.

Fallopian Tubes

The *fallopian tubes* are the tubes that connect the ovaries to the top of the uterus. Eggs travel from the ovaries through the fallopian tubes and into the uterus. Sometimes, though rarely, an egg can get embedded in one of the fallopian tubes, become fertilized, and develop there. This is called an ectopic pregnancy and must be terminated because the fetus cannot grow in the tube.

Ovaries

The *ovaries* are the two vessels where the eggs, the female's contribution to new life, are stored. A woman has all the eggs she will ever have in her two ovaries by the time she is born. Every month, as the hormones dictate, one of the ovaries will release an egg into the fallopian tube. That egg will descend to the uterus where it will either become fertilized, leading to pregnancy, or pass through the os of the uterus with the monthly menstrual blood.

Pelvic Floor Muscles

The *pubococcygeus* (PC) *muscles* make up the web of muscles that support the pelvic floor in women as well as in men. Some run front to back and others run side to side, crisscrossing to form the support system. It is these muscles that stop and start the flow of urine and bowel movements, keep the bladder from leaking, contract during orgasm, open for birthing babies, and hold the internal organs in place. Keeping these muscles toned is very important to sexual and genital health. These are the muscles that are strengthened by doing Kegel exercises.

FACT

Hormones play a big role in a woman's sexuality and her physical and emotional state before, during, and after lovemaking. If a woman has a deficiency in certain hormones, she may lose her desire for sex or notice a decrease in her libido. Hormonal changes can also affect a woman's emotional and mental state. It's important for a woman to be alert for any signs of a hormonal problem and discuss them with her doctor.

A Personal Sexology Exam

Every woman should know her body well, especially if she is interested in being powerfully erotic and sexual. A personal examination is an important first step to great sex. A personal sexology exam is usually done alone. Set aside some quality time to investigate your Jade Garden, as the ancient Chinese called a woman's vulva area.

Let's Begin Your Exploration

Start by taking a shower or bath and relaxing. If you have never done this before, view it as a way to know and love yourself better. As you relax, allow any negative imprinting, from societal or family influences or from past partners, to dissolve. Remember that many cultures have worshiped the feminine genitalia. For this moment, pretend you are a member of one of those societies and rejoice in the wondrous gifts you have been given just by being a woman!

Stand near a full-length mirror and observe your body. You're not looking at yourself critically. Rather, your attitude is one of openness, interest, reverence, and perhaps awe. Notice your hips. They have soft curves that draw the attention of potential partners. Your waistline may be smaller than your hips. Notice the softness of your skin.

Look at your breasts. No other mammal has breasts that stay full when they aren't nursing a baby. And yet, many cultures aren't as fixated on breasts as our culture is. Explore your breasts to see how they feel to your own touch and to discover how you like to be touched. You might want to use a little massage oil for this exploration.

Exploring Your Vulva

Now, find yourself a small hand mirror and sit comfortably on a mat or towel. Slowly and softly rub your hand over the pubic mound of hair between your legs. Feel how soft it is. Notice the sensations that translate through to your skin from the hair follicles. Give a slight tug to the hair with your whole hand and see how it feels when those nerve endings are stimulated more forcefully.

With both hands, gently separate the hair and open up the outer lips of your vulva. Look at the outer and inner lips in the mirror. Notice the colors and see where the hair starts and stops. See the entrance to the vagina and look for the tiny opening, just above it, that is the end of the urethra. Notice the glistening, wet skin.

Exploring Your Clitoris

Apply a small amount of lubricant to your vulva. With your thumb and forefinger, feel along both sides of your clitoris. Also explore the clitoral shaft buried just under the skin below the clitoris. You will have to squeeze your fingers together slightly to feel along the shaft. This is easier to do when you are turned on, as the shaft and head of the clitoris fill with blood and are more prominent. This is also a great stroke to use when pleasuring yourself.

Now look at and feel the hood over the clitoris. Pull it back gently to expose the head, or tip, of the clitoris. Run your finger gently over the head and feel its sensitivity. This is the most concentrated bundle of nerve endings on your whole body.

Exploring Your Vagina

With a little more lubricant, explore the inside of your vagina. At this point you may want to get up and sit on your knees. This position will give you better access to your vagina and G-spot. Feel the lining of the vaginal walls and the folds that make up the interior area.

ESSENTIAL

The Kama Sutra divides men into three categories by penis size: the Hare, the Bull, and the Horse. It also divides women into three categories of vagina size: the Deer, the Mare, and the Elephant. The perfect union is said to be between equals: the Hare man with the Deer woman, the Bull and the Mare, and the Horse and the Elephant.

As you put your finger inside your vagina, check the strength of your PC muscles by tightening on your finger. The walls should feel thick and strong. If they don't, start doing those Kegel exercises today. You'll feel improvement within a few weeks.

Where's the G-Spot?

It's difficult for women to reach their own G-spot, so you'll have to twist a little to get access to it. Your hand will probably be facing palm up, although don't hesitate to spend a little time exploring the area down toward your anus. The membrane between the anus and the vagina is thin. Because of this, the G-spot can be stimulated through the anus, too.

Just beyond the entrance to the vagina, on the top, you'll feel a mound of skin that is ridged and plump. Slip just beyond that and you've hit the G-spot area. It is neatly tucked behind the pubic bone and needs a surprisingly firm touch to be felt. It is much more responsive when you are turned on, so you may want to arouse yourself and then explore more.

When touching your G-spot, you will probably feel an area of heightened sensitivity. Touching it might even feel uncomfortable at first. You may feel slight pain, tickling, erotic sensations, or the urge to urinate. Or you may not feel much this first time. For now, just see if you can identify any spot that feels a bit more sensitive than the surrounding tissue, and just press on it or massage it for a minute or two.

Reaching the Cervix

In this position, on your knees, you may be able to feel your cervix. In some women the uterus is tipped forward, and that brings the cervix into reach. It is toward the back and is relatively large. It will feel soft and puffy. You may be able to feel the edges and the os. It may be somewhat sensitive, depending on where you are in your monthly cycle.

Some women report that they have a very sensitive turn-on area right above the cervix on the top part of the interior of the vagina. Other than this area and the G-spot, most sexologists agree that the vagina is not a particularly sensitive area. So if you ever wondered if there should be more happening in there or believed that maybe you were different, don't give it another thought.

Nevertheless, the sensitive spots you do have in your vagina are exquisite and deserve all the attention you can give them. The more you stimulate them, the more they will give back to you. This is why the angle of penetration during intercourse is so important to women.

Completing the Exercise

When you feel your exploration is complete, remove your finger and simply hold your hand softly over your vulva and mound and take a few deep breaths. Relax and appreciate yourself for this time. Honor yourself and all women. Be grateful for being given these parts that function so miraculously.

As you wrap up this time with yourself, reflect on what you thought about your private parts before you began this exercise. In particular, try to answer the following questions:

- Has your view changed?
- What did you discover?
- Do you feel more relaxed and accepting about your parts?
- Is there someone you can talk to about your discoveries and feelings? (If so, spend some time with this person talking about your experience.)

This is a fun and interesting exploration to do with your partner, too. Be vulnerable and ask him to do this with you. Then, you can switch roles so that you can watch your partner explore himself.

QUESTION

How do I figure out where my PC muscles are and how to control them? If you aren't familiar with your pelvic floor muscles, pay attention next time you pee. As you urinate, see if you can stop the flow. It's your PC muscles that are allowing you to do this.

Classic Kegel Exercises

The pubococcygeus (PC) muscle exercises known as Kegel exercises have many advantages. They are best known for their help in strengthening and toning the whole pelvic floor to prevent incontinence later in life. But they are also the secret to stronger orgasms and pompoir, the art of milking the penis during intercourse.

What is pompoir?
The art of pompoir, or milking the penis, is a marvelous technique to use with many different lovemaking positions. To perform this technique, you contract your PC muscles while the penis is inside you, simulating a milking action. Pompoir does take a while to perfect, but it is well worth it.

Doing Kegel exercises will definitely improve the sexual experience during intercourse for both you and your partner. In fact, once your PC muscles get regular exercise, you will find that pumping them actually turns you on. Furthermore, training these muscles will help you better identify and distinguish your G-spot and anal muscles.

As you perfect these exercises and strengthen the muscles, you'll begin to notice that you can isolate distinctly separate groups of muscles in your pelvic floor. This enables you to isolate your clitoris, for instance, and stimulate yourself at any time. It's an excellent trick for getting warmed up for a hot date or romantic evening.

Kegel exercises also increase blood flow to the pelvic region, which aids in the increased flow of hormones and helps engorge the vaginal area. With increased blood supply and stronger muscles, you will prep yourself for better, stronger, and more amazing orgasms.

Are You Ready to Begin?

Sit comfortably in a chair or on the floor. You should be sitting up straight, but keep a relaxed attitude. You can also use a large rolled-up towel—sit on your knees and put the towel between your legs so that you're sitting on it. You should be able to feel slight pressure on your pelvic floor.

Take a few slow, deep breaths to begin. Really relax. Breathe fully into your belly. On an in-breath, tighten your PC muscles. Hold for a moment. Now, on the out-breath, relax them. Focus on the relaxing. This is very important. Let your muscles go to a completely relaxed state. Make sure you do this after every Kegel. As you increase or decrease your speed, your breath will follow automatically. Tighten and relax, tighten and relax.

Try to start with about fifty of these every day for a few days. Your muscles may hurt a little, as in any new exercise, but that's how we know we're doing the work. Eventually, you can work up to 200 repetitions a day. You may do several sets a day, if you wish.

What Do You Notice?

You will generally notice the difference within a few weeks. After about a month, you can usually begin to isolate the different muscle groups that comprise the pelvic floor. As you continue working on your PC muscles, take notice of how they feel. Are you getting turned on just by doing the exercises? Has your partner noticed any change during intercourse?

Don't be discouraged if you don't notice much of a change right away. This will take a little time, as any muscle conditioning does, but the benefits are well worth the time and effort. You should notice that you have a better "grip" when you insert two fingers into the opening of the vagina.

Advanced Kegel Exercises

When you have mastered 200 repetitions a day and feel like your muscles have caught up to the new exercise demands you have placed on them, you can add a set of sustained Kegels to your repertoire. When you first try these, you should be sitting in a chair with your feet on the ground.

ESSENTIAL

Remember—only do what feels comfortable at any one moment. You can always come back to the exercise. Don't continue if you feel like you're hyperventilating. It will often take a little while to get into the flow of these exercises. Be gentle with yourself and enjoy them.

Begin by slowly tightening your PC muscles to the count of ten (or to whatever number you can get to when you're beginning). Hold and take one long, slow, deep belly breath and let that breath out without letting your muscles go. On the next in-breath, tighten one more time.

Begin to slowly let that breath out and let your muscles relax in a gradual letting go. Do this in steps of ten if you can—it may be very hard at first. Eventually, you can work up to twenty repetitions. You can put these into the middle or at the end of your 200 regular Kegels.

Causes for Concern

Every woman's body is unique and different. You know you own body best, especially if you've made self-exploration and examination a regular routine. Among other benefits, one good thing about this is that you will be able to quickly spot anything new or unusual. Certain fluctuations and changes are normal and expected, especially as your go through your monthly cycle. But anything that just doesn't look or feel right warrants your attention. This would include any rashes, sores, tender spots, or areas that suddenly become painful. Cysts or lumps also need to be taken seriously. Don't panic right away; many of these things can be totally normal and harmless, or easily treated. However, if it is something potential serious, the sooner you consult your doctor or seek treatment, the better off you will be.

CHAPTER 6

A Man's Body

Like women, men are rarely encouraged to know their bodies intimately or explore their full sexual potential. They may feel more permission than women to be open about their desires for sex, but that does not mean they have really explored their full capacity for passion or their deeper, subtler sensitivities. Learning about your own anatomy—how it works and how it responds to certain stimulation—can be a valuable experience for anyone, man or woman.

Male Sexuality

It's a cultural stereotype that sexuality comes naturally to men. In fact, many men feel stymied by cultural and family beliefs that stigmatize male sexuality. In many cases, a young man's sexual experiences begin with quick, furtive exploration. He may learn to reach climax quickly during masturbation. Then, when it comes to sexual excitement with a potential lover, his body may react too quickly. This pattern can be very difficult to change, leading to insecurity and fear of underperforming.

The male ego is very much tied to sexuality. Issues of acceptance, performance, attractiveness, and youthfulness really do matter for men just as much as they do for women. When you add to this the stress levels of modern life, things can get tough. Lack of good communication skills between couples and the changing roles of men and women compound the problem. Many people simply don't take the time to develop skills to be great lovers.

The Male Body

The male body is very different from the female body in terms of its reproductive organs, but new advances in medical understanding of both the male and female anatomies are revealing more similarities than differences. Modern researchers are discovering that men and women have internal and external sexual parts that are of the same origin. As the embryo develops, these parts take different developmental tracks, as directed by male and female hormones, which exist in different ratios in the male and female bodies.

Pubic Mound and Pubic Bone

Men and women both have a soft, fat-padded pubic mound, which protects the pubic bone. It is covered with hair and has scent glands that distribute pheromones, sweat, and sexual stimulus scents. The hair and hair follicles add extra erotic input by stimulating the nerve endings under the skin. Gently tugging, pulling, and scratching this area can be a turn on.

The pubic bone protects the male's internal sexual parts from outside damage. In the right positions during sex, it can be effective in rubbing against the woman's clitoris for stimulation.

Scrotum

The *scrotum* is the sac that hangs down under the penis and contains the testes and the ductwork that allows the sperm to enter the penis and be ejaculated. The skin of the scrotum is soft, pliable, and covered sparsely with hair. Some men enjoy stimulation of the scrotum during sex.

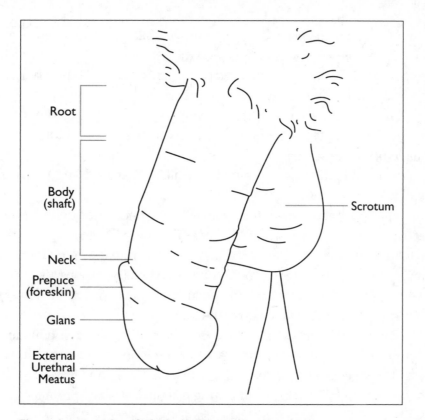

Root

Body
(shaft)

Scrotum

Neck

Prepuce
(foreskin)

Glans

External
Urethral
Meatus

The male external genitals, including penis and scrotum.

Makeup of the Penis

The penis is comprised of several parts. On the exterior, the penile skin has an amazing capacity to expand and shrink within minutes or even seconds. As the tissue underneath fills with blood, the penis goes from flaccid to erect. Blood vessels can be seen just under the skin. These become much more prominent as the erection becomes harder.

Many ancient cultures understood the sexual arts both as a science and as a spiritual path. The phallus was worshiped as a powerful creative force. These cultures bestowed names on the penis like Thunder Bolt, Wand, Jade Flute, and Arrow of Love.

At the tip of the penis is the foreskin. Just like the clitoral hood protects the clitoris, the *foreskin* covers and protects the delicate tip of the penis. If it has been removed via circumcision, the head of the penis is always exposed. The foreskin has many nerve endings and scent glands buried in it.

The penile shaft has several nerves, veins, and arteries running through it and includes the urethra, which runs through the middle. The shaft is made up of the same spongy material as the clitoral shaft—the corpus cavernosum. When this spongy material fills with blood, the penis becomes erect.

Up to one-third of the penile shaft is buried under the skin. At the other end, at the tip of the penis, is what's known as the Lowndes crown. It is buried under the tip, or head, of the penis and may be likened to the tip o f the clitoris. It is highly likely that the nerve endings here are chiefly responsible for the exquisite sensitivity of the *frenulum*, the membrane that connects the foreskin to the shaft and glans, close to the tip of the penis.

The *glans of the penis* is the very sensitive tip area. It contains a large number of nerve endings and plays a key role in male arousal. The urethra, which connects the bladder to the penis, ends here and is used for the elimination of urine; it is also used during ejaculation. Two spermatic ducts feed semen into the urethra during the ejaculation process.

At the base of the penile shaft are the two Cowper's, or bulbourethral, glands. They excrete small amounts of an alkaline fluid that neutralizes any acidity in the urine and urethral tube. This enables the sperm in the semen to travel in a favorable environment.

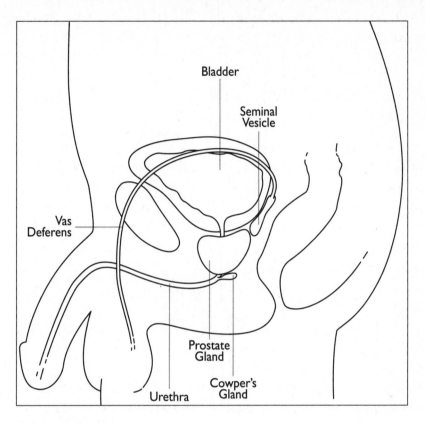

Bladder

Seminal
Vesicle

Vas
Deferens

Prostate
Gland

Cowper's
Gland

Urethra

The prostate gland.

Prostatic Glands, or the Prostate

The *prostate* is actually a group of glands clustered together at the base of the penis. The duct that delivers the sperm and the two ducts that deliver the seminal fluid all convene here, so the prostate is instrumental in male ejaculation. During ejaculation, the prostate contracts and "pumps" the fluid out through the urethra.

The prostate is thought to be the equivalent of the G-spot in the woman. When directly stimulated, it is reported to add additional heightened sensuality to a man's orgasmic experience. See Chapter 15 for more on this subject.

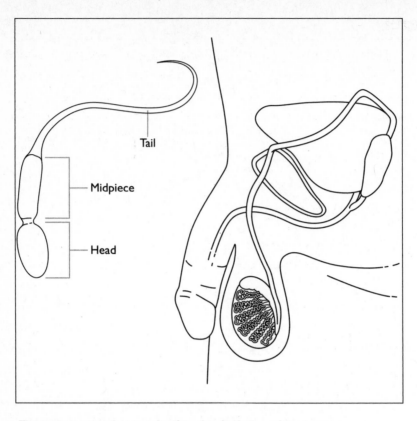

Tail

Midpiece

Head

The testes are male reproductive glands that produce sperm.

The Testes and Sperm

The *testes* are two egg-shaped glands that produce sperm. They are connected to the prostate gland, where the sperm are combined with the seminal fluids to form semen, which is then ejaculated through the vas deferens, or spermatic duct. The sperm contain the genetic material that the male contributes to fertilization. Although there are many sperm in each ejaculation, it takes just one to fertilize the egg during conception.

Prior to ejaculation, the sperm is held in seminal vesicles, sacs that hold and nourish it. The sperm bathe in a solution of simple sugar and fluids that thickens the blend until it is needed in the ejaculation process.

Perineum

The *perineum* is a soft spot on the exterior of the body, between the anus and the base of the penis (or, in the case of women, the vagina). Although it's not always apparent that this is a sexual part, the many nerve endings that surround the anus make it very sensitive. You can experience great pleasure when the perineum is pressed firmly, perhaps because it stimulates the prostate gland in men.

Kegel Exercises for Men

If you've read the chapter on the female body, you already have an introduction to Kegel exercises. Women aren't the only ones who benefit from using their PC (pubococcygeus) muscles. In fact, PC muscles are just as useful for men. They hold up the pelvic floor, hold the internal organs in the body, and generally help counteract the downward gravitational pull. Having strong PC muscles aids in stronger erections that last longer and increases libido. Kegel exercises also help massage the prostate gland.

PC muscles must be relaxed in order to urinate. They can be tightened to prevent ejaculation from occurring (although that's not necessarily the best method), and they can and should be strengthened. You can test your PC muscles by trying to use them to lift the erect penis. The higher you're able to lift your erection, the stronger your PC muscles actually are. You will notice that you can "lift" your erection a little higher when you squeeze.

FACT

The angle of the penis at the time of erection varies from man to man. Younger men tend to have angles that point upward. As men age, they tend to lose the upward swoop. This angle directly affects the stimulation of the G-spot in the woman during intercourse. Kegel exercises can strengthen the muscles that control this arc.

You can use the same Kegel exercises described in Chapter 5. A recap: first get the feeling of tightening your PC muscles by stopped your stream in mid-urination. Once you know how to squeeze these muscles, you can strengthen by repeatedly squeezing them (say, in sets of 10 or 20 reps) several times a day.

Once you feel your muscles are strengthened, you can further exercise them by using a wet washcloth or a sock draped over your erection. Lift it up and down as you are tightening and relaxing.

Does Size Really Matter?

Penis size is the subject of magazine articles, talk shows, kitchen table gossip, and locker-room whispers. As a result, many men feel self-conscious about their penis, afraid that they're just not measuring up. But the truth is, size doesn't matter—what matters is the man's self-confidence and skill. Much more important than what you've got is what you can do with it.

Becoming a wonderful, attentive, and caring lover is far more important than the size of your penis. Having a very large penis can actually be a problem. Though the vagina can expand and shrink according to fit, some vaginas are smaller than others. Difficulties can arise when two people are mismatched in this arena. A man with a larger-than-average penis may have trouble getting full satisfaction for himself because he can't penetrate deep enough to stimulate his whole shaft. Furthermore, some women complain that they experience pain from their partner's thrusting techniques, and the pain may be due to the size of the penis.

The Lock and the Key

One reason the size of a man's penis isn't very important is that the G-spot is only 1½ to 2 inches inside the vagina, and during intercourse the goal is to stimulate the G-spot to an orgasm. The head of the penis does most of the stimulating of the G-spot. As the head passes the G-spot area, on both the in- and the outstroke, it catches slightly; that's what causes stimulation. Particularly on the outstroke, the head of the penis rubs up against the pubic bone and causes friction in the G-spot area.

Women often mention that the girth of the penis is more important to them than the length. But even the girth isn't that important, as long as a woman does her Kegel exercises. With stronger PC muscles, a woman will be very satisfied with a penis of any size—and she will also have much more sexual vitality and orgasmic potential.

The Soft-On

Don't be upset if occasionally you can't get it up. There are plenty of great sexual possibilities that aren't centered around a hard-on. Take the focus off intercourse and try a side dish for a change.

When you have a soft-on, your partner may want to give you attention orally. If she usually has difficulty taking you into her mouth, now would be the perfect time. Try some new techniques and let go of performance worries. You'll enjoy yourself a lot more if you relax and go with the moment.

ALERT

The rate of prostate cancer is increasing. Having a lot of satisfying sex can help keep the prostate healthy. Vitamins, minerals, and nutrients, especially zinc, are invaluable aids in staying sexually happy and healthy. A healthy lifestyle can also help you feel your best.

A Personal Sexology Exam

Because a man's sex organs are more external than a woman's, men are more likely to have explored them. A man may know more about their capabilities and limitations than a woman does about her parts. Yet that knowledge is sometimes limited to the basics. The following exploration is suggested for you to become more intimate and connected with your body and your sexual parts.

Beginning Your Exploration

Make sure you have privacy, though you may choose to do this exercise with a partner. (If you choose to do this with a partner, make sure you take the lead. Your partner may ask questions, but the focus should be on you.) Start by taking a bath or shower and relaxing. Close your eyes and breathe for a few minutes.

Stand in front of a full-length mirror and observe your body. Look at your chest and arms. Notice how they are shaped. Don't judge yourself—simply look for the universal symbols of your maleness. Notice your hips, legs, muscles, and torso. Do you have a lot of body hair? How does it feel?

Begin by cupping your penis and scrotum in your hand and gently holding yourself. Notice the heft and feel of the weight. Where is your mind? Do your thoughts turn sexual immediately? Just breathe and relax.

Lightly pull the skin that covers your scrotum. Use both hands for this and experience the stretch and elasticity it has. Notice if your testes are the same size. Just as women's breasts are often different in size, men's testicles may be, too. Rub your hand very gently over the hair on your pubic mound. How does that feel? If a partner has touched you in that way in the past, did you like it?

Exploring Your Penis

Now, cup just your penis in one hand. If it is getting hard, relax and come back to this exercise in a minute. If you are uncircumcised, pull the foreskin forward and consider how it covers the tip and then some. Wet your fingers and gently run them around the frenulum. That's the area on the shaft of the penis just immediately below the head.

Notice the veins that are apparent on the outside of your penis, along the shaft. Now, if possible, guide yourself to an erection and look at those veins now. Notice the work they are doing to supply the blood that causes your erection. By just thinking about that blood, you may be able to pump more blood into your penis with some focus.

Arouse yourself with some of the hand techniques covered in Chapter 15, using a good-quality lubricant. Remember to focus on breathing into your belly. Then, observe yourself. What do you notice? Is your scrotum loose and relaxed or tight and up toward your body? Has its texture or color changed in any way? How does it feel to pull down gently on your scrotum as you pleasure yourself? Do you ask your lover to do this during lovemaking?

Add a bit more lubricant to your genitals and feel your scrotum again. Feel the testes in the sac. You may even be able to feel the vas deferens, the tube that delivers the sperm to the seminal vesicles. Be gentle. These are delicate parts.

Buried Treasure

Lie down. Place your hand behind and under your scrotum and feel for the base of your penis, which is buried under the skin. You should be able to grab it and even stroke it with enough lubrication. How does this feel? Can you tell if you are more sensitive on the upper area of the base or the under part?

Now, with the same hand, feel the area of your groin that is directly next to the base of your penis. This is the space that connects your legs with your torso. The next time you have sex and your lover is stimulating you, have her massage you in this area while you are aroused. If she strokes with her fingers close to the base of your shaft, it should add to the sensual feelings.

ESSENTIAL

If you'd like your partner's vagina to be tighter, don't just complain about it. Instead, tell her that you would like to practice lasting longer and suggest that she practice some of the arts of loving, too.

If you feel tight in this area, massage it without sexual arousal and practice relaxation and breathing techniques. You'll benefit from easing those muscles later, when you are engaged in lovemaking. This is very appropriate for women, too. Try it on your lover next time, as part of the foreplay.

Moving on to the Perineum

Put some light pressure in the area between the base of your penis and the anus. Press more firmly. Do you notice any sensations? It's an indirect way of stimulating the prostate gland and can feel very good when combined with heightened arousal. If you want to, lightly feel your anus around the outside. It has many nerve endings and can be highly erotic during sex. See Chapter 15 for more detailed instruction on internal prostate massage. This is a sexual secret few men or women know about.

Causes for Concern

Just as we mentioned in the previous chapter dealing with a woman's body, it's important to be alert for anything that may seem off with the private areas of your body. Anything that just doesn't look or feel right warrants your attention. This would include any rashes, sores, tender spots, or areas that suddenly become painful. Cysts or lumps also need to be taken seriously. If urination or sexually activity suddenly becomes painful or uncomfortable, this can also be a warning sign that something may be amiss. Don't panic right away—many of these things can be totally normal and harmless, or easily treated. However, if it is something potential serious, the sooner you consult your doctor or seek treatment, the better off you will be.

A sudden or drastic change in libido can also sometimes be a symptom of a medical problem, so this is something you should pay attention to, as well.

CHAPTER 7

Sexual Response in Men and Women

When you're hot, you're hot, and when you're not, you're not. Sometimes there seems to be no rhyme or reason as to what causes your sexual response (or lack thereof). Many factors determine how turned on you are at any given time—the quality of communication between partners, self-esteem, stress, feelings of warmth or closeness, family problems, stimulation or lack of stimulation, fatigue, aerobic fitness, and religious beliefs all affect your libido.

Ready or Not

You can't expect that you'll always be ready for sex. Yet many people would rather fake interest than communicate openly about their feelings. The problem with this is that it further increases the emotional distance between partners and makes great sex even less likely in the future. When you don't feel like talking much, you can simply say, "I'm not ready for lovemaking just now, but I sure would love to snuggle or spoon with you," or "I sure would love to give or receive a massage."

To help yourselves get the most out of sex, it's good to understand some things about how men and women work. Let's look at the general sexual response patterns of men and women and then expand on the possibilities.

A massage can help both men and women get into a loving mood. Some men feel they should be the macho, sexy guy who is just supposed to get it up anytime. The fact is, especially as men get older, they too need to be warmed up to enjoy sex to the fullest.

Sexual Response Curve

Sexual response in men and women can vary greatly, despite the common belief that men are always ready for sex. In reality, men need touch, desire, and attention to feel turned on, just as much as women do.

Sexual Response in Men

Men tend to be visual responders. They are stimulated by the sight of breasts, hourglass waistlines, and buttocks. When a man sees a woman walking down the street, his testosterone kicks in, and as his penis expands, his self-control shrinks. The typical male sexual response pattern unfolds like this:

1. **Excitement phase.** This can be viewed as the anticipation phase. It begins with imagining, touching, innuendo, kissing, fondling, looking at his partner, flirting, dancing, or any other activity the man finds exciting. As excitement builds, his erection hardens. On an arousal scale of one to ten, this phase takes him to about five or six.

2. **Plateau phase.** At this point, an increase in excitation occurs. The heart begins to beat faster, the erection gets firmer, the sense of separateness fades to the background, and body movements become more involuntary. The testicles and scrotum tighten and pull closer to the body. Breathing patterns can be shallow and fast. The man's excitement can escalate quickly at this point. Premature ejaculation sometimes occurs during this phase.

3. **Orgasm phase.** This is often the point of no return as the man begins to move toward orgasm and ejaculation. The penis thickens with blood and the head often swells as he gets closer to orgasm. If a man has practiced ejaculation mastery, he might be able to avoid—or at least delay—orgasm even once he has reached this point.

4. **Resolution or refractory phase.** Within minutes of ejaculation, the body relaxes, the breath deepens, and the blood begins to flow back out of the primary erogenous zones. The body comes back to its static state, before it was turned on, though much more relaxed and satisfied.

FACT

An ancient Taoist love text says that a woman's sexual energy begins in her heart and then moves to her genitals. For the man, the energy starts in the genitals and then moves to the heart. This difference, when worked with consciously, can bring about the healing of misunderstandings between men and women.

Sexual Response in Women

There's the stereotype that women take longer to get warmed up for sex than men do. This is somewhat of a myth. Part of the problem may be that women were traditionally discouraged from acknowledging or encouraging their sexual interests or desires. As a result, many women may have felt the need to deny their sexual desires and physical responses.

Another problem can occur when a woman hasn't explored her own reactions to sexual stimulation and states of physical arousal. This can lead to lots of wasted time and effort as the woman and/or her partner tries all sorts of less than successful moves and techniques in an effort to get her aroused. This can be frustrating for both people—especially for the woman, if she's only in the mood for a quickie (and yes, women often just want a quickie).

But for women who are very familiar with their bodies, not much time is needed for them be lubricated and ready. Many women reach orgasm quickly through self-stimulation but take longer to arouse and orgasm when having sex with a partner.

Regardless of individual arousal time, a woman's sexual response usually begins with feelings of emotional intimacy. She may not need such intimacy every time she makes love, but things generally go better if she feels she is getting the intimacy she needs. Tender words, touching, loving gestures, and sexual foreplay are ways to begin to warm up a woman.

As a woman becomes sexually stimulated, her chest may flush, her vulva will begin to swell, and she'll start exuding lubrication in her vagina. Her nipples may become erect and her breasts firmer. Her heart rate and breathing will speed up.

In the 1960s, sexologists Robert Masters and Virginia Johnson were the first modern doctors to research and describe in detail what we now call the female sexual response pattern. The typical female sexual response pattern looks like this:

1. **Excitement phase.** The energy builds during this first stage of sexual excitement. Vaginal tissue swells and lubrication of the membranes occurs. The supporting muscles of the pelvic floor tighten and pull upward. This expands the back of the vagina so it can accommodate the penis.
2. **Plateau phase.** The excitement response builds to a certain plateau and tends to level off. Breathing patterns can be shallow and fast, and the erogenous zones change color to brighter pinks and reds. It is during this period that tantric breathing can play an important part in increasing and sustaining the sexual feelings being generated.
3. **Orgasm phase.** The recognition that orgasm will occur has a distinct beginning. Many women feel this moment coming only to experience it fading and then returning. That pattern may occur several times before the orgasm phase moves into its final release. Many women experience frustration at this juncture and find that the actual orgasm may be elusory. If the orgasm does come, a very pleasurable explosive release of

pulsating energy occurs. There may be multiple phases of pulsating explosion and release.

4. **Resolution or refractory phase.** The body relaxes, the breath deepens, and the blood begins to flow back out of the primary erogenous zones. The body comes back to its static state, before it was turned on, though it is much more relaxed and satisfied. For some women this phase will last for just a few moments; others will feel complete and won't want to be aroused again for some period of time. In fact, the clitoral area is very sensitive for some women at this point and stimulation may be uncomfortable or even painful for a short time until they have a chance to recover.

Experiencing Multiple Orgasms

Many men experience multiple orgasms when they are in their twenties, and these almost always include ejaculation. As men enter their thirties, though, changes begin to occur. The refractory phase lasts longer in older men because it takes longer for the penis to refill with blood after a first orgasm with ejaculation. Men can learn to shorten this refractory phase or they can try to achieve orgasm without ejaculation.

In women, multiple orgasms can be defined several ways. The orgasms can be back-to-back responses that have distinct beginnings and ends, or they can be so close that it doesn't feel like any refractory period has occurred.

During extended multiple orgasms experienced by a woman, constant waves of involuntary muscle contractions occur. As the vaginal walls contract, the vaginal fit usually gets tighter. Rather than diminishing the woman's sexual energy, multiple orgasms often get successively more intense.

Multiple orgasms trigger a series of peaks and dips in pleasure. Each peak is higher than the one before; each dip is a period of rest, but the body does not enter a typical refractory or resolution period.

A Variety of Ways to Extend the Sexual Response Cycle

Back-to-back orgasms can occur through clitoral, G-spot, or vaginal stimulation. Typically, if a woman were able to have several clitoral orgasms in a row, they would occur with a distinct beginning and end with a fairly short refractory phase. She would be ready to go again very quickly and could take clitoral stimulation again, though she may have to start very softly the second time around.

In the case of G-spot or vaginal orgasms, they can occur like clitoral ones where the response cycle is repeated in its entirety, or the orgasms could be indistinguishable from one another. There would be no refractory period and the orgasmic state would simply continue—often being experienced as successively more intense rather than diminishing.

Take Yourself into a State of Bliss

Some women report sustaining a state of orgasmic bliss without dips for several hours. While this may be surprising, these are women who have learned to do this through practicing the exercises that are presented in this book. A woman can train herself to experience great amounts of pleasure. This is something any woman can do—with sufficient motivation and focused attention.

To facilitate becoming multiorgasmic, practice the deep-breathing exercises suggested in this book. Also, learn to drive, or enable, your orgasms by consciously increasing the pace of your breathing. A great pattern is to pant into your belly eight to ten times and then take a deep breath in and let it out very slowly through slightly pursed lips. Focus on feeling erotic pleasure in and around your genitals when doing this breathing practice. Repeat as often as you want.

Mastery over Ejaculation

Tantrics and Taoists practice ejaculation control techniques that are said to allow the chi, or life force energy, to build in a man as he ages. The teachers of these practices today say that a man may have orgasms but should retain his semen, to increase his energy and sexual drive. These techniques take some practice, but in most cases, you are almost guaranteed results if you or you and your partner are willing to learn them.

It often takes just a few weeks to become proficient. You'll last a lot longer and your lover will feel the benefits, too. Within a month you should actually be able to feel the orgasmic sensations without ejaculation and the loss of fluid. You'll feel much more energized and sexually alive instead of depleted after sex. (Specific techniques for holding your sexual charge longer are covered in Chapter 14.)

FACT

In 2000, Tantra.com surveyed 1,377 men about their control over ejaculation. The survey revealed that 20 percent ejaculate earlier than they would like to, 35 percent have control over when they ejaculate, and another 45 percent only have control some of the time.

Now that you are aware of the basic structure of the orgasmic response cycle, you can visualize what is possible. Keep this in mind when you need a little help in self-control. Very soon your body will know the difference and your leap of faith will be rewarded.

As you advance in these practices, you'll begin to notice that you are actually getting so close to the edge that you are experiencing orgasmic sensations over and over. Waves of orgasms and energy can flood your body. As you begin to have multiple orgasms, you'll notice that your penis will be anywhere from very hard to firmly soft. You can go on and on without the refractory period.

Enhancing the Female Orgasm

There are several ways in which women can enhance their orgasms, whether they're clitoral, vaginal, or G-spot orgasms. The clitoral orgasm is arguably the easiest to achieve. As a woman becomes more stimulated and turned on, the shaft and crura of the clitoris become engorged with blood. As this happens, the shaft straightens out and becomes erect, much like a penis. In the process, the head of the clitoris actually becomes more buried under the clitoral hood. This can become a problem if the woman maintains a body pose that tightens and curls inward as she becomes more turned on. The clitoris tends to get further buried. Learn to relax your body and even arch your back, slightly, if you feel this might be the case.

Some women have learned to facilitate access to the clitoral tip by pulling back the clitoral hood. Usually this will happen after a woman is somewhat turned on already. As she needs more stimulation, she will help expose her clitoral tip, either during oral sex or with finger stimulation.

The Clock Exercise

The clock exercise is a very important exercise that is rarely taught. Try it by yourself or with a partner.

Lie on your bed with your partner at your side. On your back, spread your legs open wide and relax. Take in a few deeply relaxing breaths. Now, as your partner watches, take your index finger, with a lot of lubrication on it, and feel your clitoris gently on all four sides. Now, notice if one area or side feels more excitable than another.

You'll be interested to know that on most women, if you use the analogy of a clock, the 10:00 or 2:00 positions on their clitoris are by far the most sensitive. Most women don't know this. It's such a tiny area that most women think that the nerve bundle covers the whole thing. Not true. You will most likely be much more sensitive at one of these points than the other.

FACT

In a 2009 *Redbook* survey, 51 percent of the female respondents said they reach an orgasm always or almost always during sex with their partner. Also, 35 percent said they never fake orgasms. Of those who do, 60 percent said they do it to spare their partner's feelings, while about a third said they do it in order to wrap up the sexual encounter.

When you have found which part of the clitoris is most sensitive for you, have your partner touch you softly so that you can guide him to the exact spot. As you move into oral sex, make sure you are in a position that actually focuses on this area. After you have tried the exercise and explored the sensitive areas of your clitoris, take note when you are making love to determine if you are getting the most direct stimulation you can.

G-spot Clues

Women can also achieve orgasm through stimulation of the G-spot. The more you explore the G-spot and focus on it as part of your sexual experience, the more alive and responsive it will become. At first, some women will experience burning sensations, the urge to urinate, mild pain, or possible numbness. Some women will feel like laughing or crying, or they'll feel waves of emotion. Some will experience sexual pleasure immediately. If you don't experience pleasure right away, take the view that you have at least taken a step on the path to ecstasy. If it feels like a struggle in the beginning, take breaks, but keep exploring. With time and patience, you'll get to the pleasure you're seeking.

Be gentle with yourself the first few times. Don't make it a chore. As you become more aware of your sensitive vaginal parts, you'll begin to notice how much you can feel during intercourse. The more you can feel, the more pleasure you'll have, and the more you will take control of your orgasmic response.

Do your Kegel exercises. This can't be stressed enough. They are vitally important because they give you the ability to feel what is going on inside your body. They put you in touch with the interior of your vagina and strengthen your body's response to sexual pleasure.

Female Ejaculation

Until recently, many women have felt ashamed or embarrassed about exuding fluid during sex, but public opinion has changed. Now women tend to feel that the ability to ejaculate gives them a sense of erotic power or a sense of freedom. As more women talk to each other openly about sex, they have empowered themselves to feel good about whatever feels natural and pleasurable.

Ejaculating can be somewhat messy, and it is certainly not necessary for great sex, so it's important to know that it isn't strange or unusual. If you have experienced ejaculation, you might want to be prepared with a towel next to the bed. Some women have been known to ejaculate up to several teaspoons of fluid.

The fluid emitted is exactly like male ejaculate, only without the sperm. It is not urine, though because the ejaculate comes through the urethral tube, it may push out a small amount of urine prior to the release of the ejaculate. Considering that the fluid most often occurs through G-spot or vaginal stimulation, and that the G-spot is the urethral sponge or female prostate gland, this makes perfect sense.

As in the male, the fluid in the female prostatic gland builds up and needs release. Some believe that symptoms of PMS might be greatly alleviated by female ejaculation. Part of the pressure and fluid buildup during the menstrual period may very well be female ejaculate. If you have PMS and know the times of the month when you feel the symptoms the most, have a lot of sex just prior to these times—it may help.

What's Normal, What's Not

Many people often question whether their sexual arousal and level of interest is normal. They may wonder if they are too slow to warm up or, on the other hand, if they reach the point of climax too quickly. Once again, this is something that varies widely from one person to another. Don't try to compare yourself to others. For one thing, you can drive yourself crazy trying to figure out how you stack up against other people. Not to mention, you can't be sure you are getting totally accurate information. It probably won't shock you to learn that many people lie or exaggerate their sexual stats.

ESSENTIAL

Don't be afraid to talk to your doctor about libido issues and other sexual problems. She has heard it all before. Besides, this could be a sign of an underlying medical condition. If your doctor seems uncomfortable or unwilling to discuss these types of issues, you may need to look for a doctor who is more receptive to discussing your concerns.

The important thing is figuring out what's normal—and ideal—for you. If you experience a sudden or drastic change in your libido or your ability to become sexually aroused, try to figure out what might be causing it. Red flags include: inability to become sufficiently aroused (meaning, inability to maintain an erection for men or inability to become lubricated and/or engorged for women), inability to reach a climax even after sufficient stimulation, and premature climax. Unfortunately, lots of things can disrupt your ability to become aroused or reach a climax, including medical conditions, prescription medications, and illness or injury. The good news: many of these situations are temporary or can be easily remedied.

However, should you notice a sudden change in your sexual responses that occurs for no apparent reason, you might want to address it with your doctor. It's possible there's a medical cause. (If not, you might need to consider whether it could be caused by a physiological or emotional issue, such as a problem with your relationship.) Keep in mind that slight fluctuations in desire and arousal are totally normal. For women, this often follows a pattern according to their menstrual cycle.

Sexual Dysfunction in Men

Although many sexual problems exist among both sexes, there are several dysfunctions specific to each gender. Common issues that face men include guilt about sexual desires and the pressure to perform. A good sexologist who is trained in sexuality problems may be able to help you overcome persistent problems.

Psychological problems with libido, fast ejaculation, not ejaculating, and attaining and maintaining erections often point to the presence of guilt, shame, unfulfilled desire, poor communication, or lack of training. It's amazing what happens when a couple begins to talk honestly about their anxieties, worries, and assumptions around sexual issues. The improvement can be immediate—and impressive.

Health plays an integral role as well, and factors that lead to problems with libido and erections may be physiological. These can often be treated very effectively with diet changes, herbal formulas, and smoking cessation. Overindulgence in food, smoking, or alcohol causes blood vessels to close down, which leads to lack of adequate blood flow to the penis.

If your efforts do not meet with instant success, don't be discouraged. You are not alone. This is a path that has been traveled by many men over many centuries. With an open mind and a willing heart, you can accomplish anything. For many people the most difficult hurdle to overcome is just getting started. Once you begin, you may be surprised at the rich rewards awaiting your efforts.

Sexual Dysfunction in Women

For women, overcoming and transforming problems with orgasmic potential can feel daunting at times. Learning to relax your body can help you learn to relax your mind. This will help take off some of the pressure.

Sit down and have a really good conversation about your beliefs, struggles, inhibitions, and frustrations with your lover. Be vulnerable and tell your partner your innermost feelings. Lack of communication is the number-one cause of libido problems, so stop beating yourself up and start expressing yourself more. For a little while, have sensual times together that aren't necessarily sexual or don't involve intercourse. Receiving a massage and snuggling together are the kinds of things can help take the worry out of being close.

ESSENTIAL

As you receive the massage, don't expect to end up having sex. Explore your erogenous zones fully. Be touched and learn not to do anything about it except moan. Let your lover know that in learning to receive, you are taking action, and, if he is patient, you will both see great results.

Drop the focus on the big O for a while. Be sensual. Learn to relax and receive. If you are willing, have your partner blindfold you and give you a sensual massage. The blindfold will add a little suspense and newness and will allow you to focus more fully on sensations.

Educate yourself about your own body. Spend as much time as you can learning what works best for you and what feels great. Experiment. Don't hold back. You have nothing to lose and everything to gain. You are in charge of your pleasure.

If you find yourself totally unable to reach any type of arousal, don't have sex just because you feel guilty or obligated. It's better to be honest with your partner (while stressing that you are still very attracted to them). For women especially, having sex when you aren't physically aroused can be uncomfortable or even painful—not to mention frustrating and unfulfilling.

If you really feel stuck, visit a doctor of sexology or a psychologist with a sexuality background. You'll learn a lot and discover that you aren't alone.

They will have a variety of ideas that, when combined with what you've learned in this chapter, will give you new tools for attaining your maximum pleasure potential.

Jumpstart a Lagging Libido

Recognize Your Sexiness

Many of us go through periods where we feel like the least sexy person on the planet. This is especially true for women with young kids, who may spend much of their time in Mommy clothes and are often lucky if they can shower on a daily basis. Remind yourself that you are a sexy creature, even if you may not look like it all the time. If you are feeling a bit drab, treat yourself to a bubble bath or a trip to a salon. At the very least, get your partner to watch the kids while you take a decent shower and indulge in a little personal grooming.

Self-Exploration and Self-Stimulation

Maybe you've simply gotten tired of doing the same old thing in the bedroom. By experimenting when you are alone and can take your time, you might discover that you enjoy unusual sensations or new moves. You may even discover a few erogenous zones you never knew you had!

Spice Things Up

Again, it's common to get all hot and bothered if things have gotten boring in the bedroom. Shake things up by trying something different. Experiment with adult toys, engage in some role-playing, add a few props or costumes, or watch some erotic movies with your partner. Sometimes even a little change can make a big difference.

Try Some New Sensations

Adding some gels, lotions, or massage oils can help kickstart your body's own natural lubrication. Some oils and lotions are even heat-activated or flavored and can really spice up your sexual encounters.

CHAPTER 8

Setting the Stage

The whole world is a stage, but you and your partner will probably be staging most of your plays in the bedroom. Creating an erotic atmosphere that is conducive to your unique style of romance can be a fun activity that the two of you can do together. The mood you set in your bedroom and your home guides the energy and expands your awareness of lovemaking with your partner.

Rekindling Romance

Setting the stage starts with romance—the little things two people can do any time of the day or night to communicate, "I love you. . . . I want you. . . . I'm glad I'm with you. . . . I'm looking forward to being intimate with you." The word romance means different things to different people. In a sense, it's whatever turns you on.

ESSENTIAL

People feel more romantic when they feel valued. We all want to be appreciated and acknowledged. That's really all that romance is about. There's nothing mystical or difficult to get. Just hold your partner in your thoughts, and the little gestures will follow.

The Little Gestures

Just in case romantic little gestures don't come to you automatically, make yourself a list of some of the simple things you could do to let your lover know you find him attractive or to make life a little nicer for that person. Smile when your partner comes into the room. Listen to his stories. Make the bed in the morning. Do the things that are out of the ordinary for you. Open the door for your partner. Cook a meal or do the laundry without being asked. Take the dog for a walk, mow the lawn, or clean the garage. It is amazing how much benefit comes from these actions.

Romantic Moments

Create romantic moments as you move through your day together. Americans don't display public affection nearly as much as many other cultures do, but there are things that are certainly appropriate even in our culture. Take hold of the hand next to yours when you are walking. Kiss in public. Play childlike romantic games during the day with each other—play footsies under the table or cover your lover's eyes with your hands while sitting down for a meal.

The Great Getaway

Get away to another world. Go for a mini-holiday to a local hideaway. Take all the things you think you might need for a complete getaway that heals and nourishes your bodies and spirits. This might mean going out into nature, or it may be a weekend in the big city. Whatever you choose, you will both remember it for a long time if you pack the few things that will help the memories last.

Ambiance in the Bedroom

The bedroom helps set the mood when you awake in the morning, and it's your last sense of place at night when you go to sleep. To help keep you at your best, create a space that is sensual, spicy, cozy, and private. Your bedroom can be a sanctuary and a hideaway where you start and end your day.

By creating beauty, harmony, and a clean functional space in which to enjoy our sensual and sexual life, you feed your spiritual side as well as your esthetic needs. Living harmoniously with the energy of the surrounding environment is an art form.

Feng Shui in the Bedroom

There is a way of harmonizing two peoples' energies using the ancient art of *feng shui* (pronounced *fung schway*). Feng shui is defined as the Chinese art and science of placement for arranging buildings, objects, and space in an environment in order to achieve the most harmonious balance of energy.

The idea in using feng shui in your bedroom is to blend masculine and feminine energies and create an atmosphere of trust, openness, and oneness between the two. Arranging the energy, or chi, of the room can create harmonization in the bedroom. Your last impressions before falling asleep will filter into your unconscious mind and set the stage for a restful sleep. And what you see upon opening your eyes is your first impression that sets the stage for your relationship to the new day. Does your bedroom welcome you back into consciousness, or are you smacked with overwhelming messages like laundry spilling out of the closet, unread books crowding your bedside table, and unpleasant news in old newspapers on the floor?

In studying the feng shui of the bedroom, we see that the placement of the bed, the availability of light and air, and the flow that is created in the room are important aspects to keep in mind. You may want to consider the colors you have chosen and the comfort level that you desire. Is the room inviting? How does its energy feel to you and your partner?

Make a shift in the position of the bed. If possible, avoid placing the bed directly across from the door or on a wall adjacent to bathroom plumbing. Create a cozy eddy by placing the bed to the side of the room where it still has a view of the door. Put desks and exercise equipment into another room; if they must stay, use a standing screen or curtain to separate them when they aren't in use.

The Four Elements

The four elements are earth, air, fire, and water, and having a balance of all these elements in your bedroom will help you harmonize its energy. The element earth might be a piece of driftwood you found or a stone that has special meaning to you. Living plants—either freshly cut flowers or potted plants—with rounded, soft leaves, are also a welcome addition to the bedroom.

Air becomes visible when we light incense. Fire is visible when we light a candle. Water might be represented by a small fountain or by a picture with the element water in it—but you should avoid turbulent seascapes and fountains that may become mildewed.

The Use of Color

Sometimes just small changes can make big differences. Try a change of color to set a different mood. Creamy tones combined with shades of pinks, oranges, reds, and browns help create a warm atmosphere. Pure whites, blues, and greens are cooler colors that don't have the warmth and passion usually associated with sexuality. When you can, use natural fabrics like cotton and wool for the bedding and floors. Natural fibers are friendlier to the skin, since they breathe better. They also tend to be more sensual.

Mirror on the Wall

You may also want to add a mirror to an appropriate place on a wall or on the ceiling; if it is on the ceiling, make sure it is not made of glass, for safety reasons. Mylar can be a good substitute for glass, since it is not breakable; and it gives an interesting impressionistic aura to the images it reflects. From a feng shui point of view, however, large mirrors are not advised in the bedroom because they affect the free flow of chi.

Background Music

Can you imagine a great movie without the accompaniment of an emotionally evocative soundtrack? Researchers have found that the pleasure centers of the brain that are positively stimulated by food and sex are also affected by music. Any music that sends chills up your spine has a direct effect upon your mood. When we use music that is particularly stimulating to us in a positive way, we can elevate our mood to feel more content, relaxed, energized, or turned on.

A Soundtrack to Love

You wouldn't want to leave music out of a great night of lovemaking. Music helps set the mood and can even be used to choreograph an evening of love. You probably have your old favorites, songs and artists that really turn you on and that you and your partner have made love to before. Great! Use them, but also go out and find some music that is new to both of you. You may even want to make a date to go to a music store and listen to a variety of new and different kinds of music.

Listen to new music before you introduce it to the bedroom. Explore unusual possibilities that might include world beats, drums, and exotic cultural music. Introducing new rhythms will open up the two of you to spontaneously trying new positions and practices that wouldn't have occurred to you before.

Try creating a whole playlist of music to make love to. This could be for a special erotic evening that may be several hours long. It could be a soundtrack you use for massage dates. Or it could include a hotter, spicier list of tunes that you use when you're feeling especially daring.

The idea of creating your own soundtrack allows you to create the "dance" you want. It can start with soft, melodic pieces that slowly rise in intensity, according to the length and love rhythm you and your partner share. Maybe you are creating a special birthday ritual and you want to design a new wave of lovemaking that is a gift to your beloved.

ALERT

You can find virtually any type of music imaginable online. Searching for an obscure album or a particular song from years ago? Perhaps you'd like to surprise your partner with the song your two first danced to. Odds are, with a little online searching, you'll be able to locate even the most unusual song.

At the end of the music mix, include a soft, sensuous ending when you can cuddle, kiss, and take in each other's breath before falling off to dreamland, or before getting up and continuing your day. But whatever you do, be sure to close your lovemaking sessions tenderly and sensitively.

Fragrance and Aromas

Scents and aromas are powerful stimuli; they can affect your mood and trigger memories or particular feelings. Our emotional body stores and recalls events in our lives that often have a smell or particular scent associated with them. We all experience times when we catch a scent of something that reminds us of a childhood experience, a first love, or a favorite holiday.

Researchers have found that certain foods with strong odors cause penile blood flow to increase. Dr. Alan R. Hirsch tested thirty scents and forty-six odors with men from ages eighteen to sixty-four. His results found that cinnamon buns caused the greatest arousal and that a combination of pumpkin pie and lavender caused an average increase in penile blood flow of 40 percent. Older men responded more to vanilla and men who had the best sex lives reported a preference for the aroma of strawberries. Every scent and odor that was used in the research caused some degree of increase in penile blood flow.

FACT

Dr. Hirsch also studied female reactions, which turned out to be markedly different. Among women between the ages of eighteen and forty, licorice was the most sexually stimulating. The combination of licorice and cucumber caused a 13 percent increase in vaginal blood flow. The pumpkin and lavender combination that the men liked so well caused an 11 percent increase. Women had negative responses to barbecue smoke, which caused a 14 percent decrease, and cherry, which caused an 18 percent decrease. In addition, women had a 1 percent decrease in vaginal blood flow when they were exposed to a variety of men's colognes!

Experiment with Scents

Humans can detect between 10,000 and 30,000 different scents, so have fun experimenting to find the ones that get you and your partner going. Get a variety of essential oils from a local herb shop or health food store and use them in different ways. Try putting a few drops on the light bulb in the lamp next to your bed. Bring a bowl of fruit to bed with you and try feeding tiny pieces to each other. Before you put the bites in your lover's mouth, inhale their sweet scent and let your lover do the same. You may want to blindfold your partner to really enhance the senses of taste and smell.

Attire in the Bedroom

Costuming and erotic wear have seen many changes over time. From extremely suggestive bustiers that pushed up the breasts and tightened the waist to voluminous fabric and veils that revealed very little skin, the designs tended to fit the culture and times. Today, in the privacy of our own homes, we find it a little easier to let our imaginations go wild.

Although eventually you'll end up nude, foreplay can become much more powerful and extended when you add the element of clothing. Certain clothing elements lend themselves to the erotic.

Buttocks, breasts, legs, and shoulders (in that order) are the body parts that men list as their most arousing. Therefore, plunging necklines, tight skirts, and styles that accentuate the legs, stockings, and bare shoulders are evocative ways in which women can create allure. For the bedroom, try looser-fitting garments that allude to the curves of the body underneath the clothing. The fabric should wrap around you to accentuate your own erotic, natural curves.

The Bare Essentials

It only takes a few items to satisfy a hunger for erotic dressing up. You can keep it as simple as this:

- A sarong made from either rayon or silk (to be worn by both men and women)
- A sarong that is either transparent or see-through
- A teddy, matching bra, and underwear, or a one-piece body suit
- A robe of velvet, silk, or rayon
- A feather boa

In addition, you could add any number of items that appeal to you and your partner. You can use the following list of items if you're looking for an erotic gift for your partner:

- Additional scarves of all sorts
- Dress-up items from used clothing stores
- Fantasy items that you think might be good additions to your love play
- A wider selection of lacy underwear and teddies
- Feathery fans, masks, and other props that might add appeal
- Jewelry that lends an exotic feel to your costumes

Choose fabrics like velvet, rayon, and silk—they feel just as good to the person wearing them as to the one touching them. Silk slides under the hand and over the body easily. It shimmers and feels slinky and gives the body a moist, wet look.

Erotic Clothing for Men

Though it's usually women that we think of as dressing in erotic attire, men have a few options available, too. In studies, women say they appreciate inner strength and caring in a man over physical traits, but when it comes to the physical, they list average build, tight stomachs, and strong arms as their preference. Select silk robes, boxer shorts, and maybe a sarong for your intimate liaisons. For a special evening, you may even want to layer a little and put on a pair of men's G-string underwear under your boxers. When selecting items that create a tighter look with the bulges in all the right places, pick fabrics that will breathe and that aren't too restrictive. It's a well-known fact that a man's sperm count goes down when his scrotum is up close to his body for long periods of time. Select items that leave your whole body available for touching.

ESSENTIAL

Learning to wrap and wear a sarong is quite convenient for those moments when you are undressed and need to get up for something you've forgotten. It may even come in handy when you decide to create an erotic dance for your partner some evening.

Nothing Like a Hot Bath

There is nothing like a hot bath to invigorate both your mind and your body. A hot bath can inspire you to relax and stop thinking. It can calm you and create an atmosphere of sanctuary. Taking a bath is a ritual that is easy to do for yourself.

The act of bathing together can be as elaborate or as simple as you'd like to make it. It's easy to add bubbles to the bath water and light a few candles around the bathtub. Or you can get as elaborate as using a Japanese dry brush to pamper and stimulate the skin before you get into the water. Sometimes it's appropriate to bring music, drinks, food, and playful fantasy into the bath. Other times you may want to ceremoniously wash your partner's feet and anoint them with creams and oils. You can even have an important conversation while soaking in the bathtub.

There is no end to the imaginative things you can do in the bath. Get innovative and think up a few wild ideas for yourself. Here are a few suggestions of things to do in the bath:

- Lovingly wash your partner's hair
- Give your partner a foot or scalp massage
- Slide your soapy body up and down over your partner's body
- Put soap on a large soft sponge and soap your partner's body
- Dry your partner very lovingly
- Brush each other's hair

You may also want to add something to the bath water for an enhanced experience. Here are a few ideas:

- Put rose petals in the bath and on the floor of the bathroom
- Use a few drops of a favorite essential oil in the bath
- Use herbal and scented soaps
- Finely grate a little orange or lemon rind into the tub
- Float a cinnamon stick or a few cloves in the water
- Use foaming bath bubbles

Arranging for Worry-Free Time

It's very important to have the peace of mind required for an erotic evening. What keeps men and women distracted are the regular old things that consume our everyday life—work, deadlines, laundry, company coming, kids, and almost anything else that worries us.

Clear the space as best you can, and then don't worry about what you're not doing. All of that stuff will eventually get done, whether you worry about it or not. The difference will be that you will be much more relaxed and happy. You may even find that when you give yourselves pleasurable evenings to remember, you are more resilient in handling the stresses of your daily lives.

ESSENTIAL

Something as simple as moving to another part of your house can often provide enough of a change to make things exciting. You might be surprised at the different sensations you feel just by lying on or against walls, counters, or furniture outside of your bedroom. (On the downside, you may never look at your rec room the same way again!)

Time Away from the Kids

If you have children, try to find friends or relatives to take them for an evening and overnight, if possible. Explore trading this gift with another couple by having each other's children overnight. As time passes and your children get older, you'll get better at carving out time for you and your partner. They'll understand that the two of you want time together and that you need your privacy. In the meantime, set up situations that eliminate the worry and distraction that can occur in a busy household.

CHAPTER 9

Fun with Foreplay

Almost anything done at any time might fall into the category of foreplay, as long as it's pleasurable. There are so many ways to give and receive pleasure. Every person and every couple is different. So why not include anything that has ever been associated with pleasure over your whole lifetime in your expanded definition of foreplay? A great definition might be everything right up to intercourse! Sometimes it's appropriate and exciting to just have fun with foreplay and skip the main course. Explore and have a good time.

Foreplay Twenty-Four Hours a Day

It's very erotic to feel loved and cherished. Do you remember the first time you were in love? You probably couldn't stop thinking about your heart-throb. That was nonstop foreplay.

Mature couples usually need a little help to remember that it's important to think of your partner during the day, when you are not in each other's presence. Call your partner to say you are thinking of her. Both men and women love even the smallest gestures that show they are in someone's heart.

ALERT

Don't underestimate the power of extended foreplay! If you have a fulfilling sex life, you might think you don't need to extend the warm-up phase. But this can be the most enjoyable part of lovemaking. Many couples find that foreplay provides them with some of their most pleasurable sexual moments. So don't skimp on the foreplay!

Inquire about your lover's schedule, and ask often how he is doing. Ask if there is anything you can help with. Pack a little note in your lover's briefcase, purse, or lunch pail to be found during the day. Hint at a secret meeting later that evening. Tease a little. Touch each other often.

Of course, the standard things work well, too: flowers, dinner out, a movie, a gift—all are usually welcomed and appreciated. But those things aren't nearly as important as the little remembrances that don't cost much. When you can offer help and assistance, that is foreplay. When you say "I love you" in many different ways—you are having foreplay. And these things are not just for men to do and for women to receive. They are important for both sexes.

Erotic Massage

Massage is a practice that has been perfected over thousands of years. It is used for stress reduction, relaxation, erotic touch, musculature health, lymphatic health, emotional release, body rebalancing, and much more.

When we daydream of the perfect sensual experience with a lover, it often includes massage. Nothing can get a couple more relaxed, in the moment, and focused than warm oil and tender hands. Massage is a wonderful way to begin a sexual experience. It gets our bodies and our minds in tune for what comes next.

One of the basic things to keep in mind when giving a massage is to prepare ahead. Where will you give the massage—on the bed, on a massage table, or possibly in front of the fire? When you decide, make sure you have a large-enough towel or an old sheet. You don't want to use oil on or near anything new or valuable.

Warm the massage oil slightly. Get your music selection ready. Warm the room ahead of time. If you are prepared, your participant will feel even more honored to receive this gift.

Begin Massaging Your Lover's Body

When you are ready, have your lover lie down on his stomach. Invite him to relax and receive your love and energy. Ask if there is anything he needs before you begin.

To start, rub your hands together vigorously for a couple of minutes to get them warm and energized. Tenderly place them on your partner's back and let them just lie there for a few minutes as you connect.

Lightly move your hands in slow, smooth motions over your lover's body. Feel your fingers and palms. Do they feel good? Make whatever adjustments you need to make so that you, the giver, feel comfortable and relaxed, and so that your hands are receiving pleasure as well as giving it. Feel the soft hair on your lover's body. Feel the lines and contour of his calves, thighs, buttocks, waist, back, neck, and arms.

Oil Massage

Apply some warm oil or massage lotion to your hands and begin with the feet. At this point you can use firmer pressure, but remember that sensual massages aren't therapeutic in nature! You are eroticizing the flesh, not pounding it.

Massage the balls of the feet along with the instep, heel, and ankle. Go between the toes and on top of the arch. Send love through your hands to heal and nurture. Move up the leg and spend a little time on the calves, behind the knees, and on the thighs. It's best to work on one side and then the other.

ALERT

> Try not to make your partner flinch during a massage. Experiment with the depth and pressure of the touch you give. Start with a lighter touch and move into deeper pressure later. Stay sensitive to your partner's response and adjust accordingly.

Move to the torso and gently knead the buns. As you apply new oil, try leaving one hand on your partner and pouring a little oil over the hand that is still on the body. This serves two purposes; it keeps your partner from being shocked by the oil and it keeps you and your lover connected. Your lover won't feel like you've gone away, even for a minute. Try moving your hands in unison over his bottom. Go in circles, first one way and then the other way. This is relaxing and energizing all at the same time. Ask how he likes it best—whether he wants your touch to be deeper or lighter.

Moving On

As you move up the torso, you can use more oil. Slowly work up the spine, but never touch it directly. The muscles on either side of the spine support and protect the vertebrae and the rib attachment points. See if you can feel every one of them as you move slowly up the back. You'll find that using your thumbs will work well. As you continue the massage, make sure that your fingers and hands are doing fine and aren't tired or uncomfortable. Remember, this experience should be pleasant for both you and your lover.

Move to the outer area of the back and run your hands up the sides of the body, from the waist to the armpits. Use a long, firm stroke so you don't tickle. Keep your attention focused on the sensations in your hands. There are lots of nerve endings in this region and it can be a major erogenous zone for many people. Spend some time on the shoulders and scapula.

As you work these areas, you can move a little closer and tease your partner with a little verbal foreplay. Tell him how much you're enjoying this moment or anything that comes to mind. Or just plant a simple kiss on the back of his neck.

Finish the sides by massaging each arm and the hands. Our hands serve us well and they get cramped and tired. You can kiss them and knead them lovingly and even speak to them and thank them for all the service they perform. Experiment using both hands to work up and down the arm, or hold the hand firmly with one of your hands and massage up the arm with your other hand. This allows for gentle pulling and stretching of the arm.

Face Up

Gently role your partner over and connect with your eyes for a few moments. Though you can do his feet again, you may want to begin with the front of his legs and thighs. Try moving your hands out from the middle, at the knee, up with one hand to the thigh and down with the other hand toward the toes. You can also stand at his feet and move both of your hands up each leg in unison.

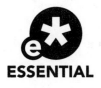

ESSENTIAL

If the massager is a woman, she can use her breasts in the massage. As she reaches toward her lover's inner thigh, her breasts can grace his feet. The breasts are the representation of the heart and can be used to send her love.

The inner thighs are highly erotic areas that generally respond immediately to soft, conscious touch. Notice your partner's breath as you approach this area. Did he make a satisfied sigh? Did he moan?

You may want to encourage your partner to open his legs a little now. The muscle structure of the inner thighs is sensitive, so use a soft stroke. Lightly play with his pubic hair and really feel the soft hair on his thighs. Hair is highly erotic, and the more softly you can touch it the better it will feel. Gently brush over his genitals, just teasing a little, and move to the front of the torso.

Add more oil and massage the belly and abdomen with the palms of your hands. Be firm but sensitive, especially if your partner has eaten in the last few hours. Then move on to the chest area.

As you move up the body, start in the center, move up between the breasts, and stroke to the outside and around the breasts. Include the upper chest and come down around the outside of the breasts and back down. Start the move again. This is a particularly good massage move to open the heart area. Do it a few times with your attention focused on love. You may even want to speak loving words to your partner.

Now, focus some attention on the breasts. Women generally love having their breasts massaged upward and on the outsides, under their arms. Use circle strokes, first one way, six times, and then the other. Massage the areola and nipples gently. Men's breasts can be highly sensitive, too. Focus some attention on them to develop their erotic potential even more.

Finish the main body massage by standing at your partner's head and massaging his shoulders and arms from this position. Knead the muscles in the shoulders and stretch your body over your partner's, using both of your arms to massage down his arms to his hands. Women, as you bend with this move, let your breasts lightly brush your partner's face. Repeat this stroke several times.

A Facial Massage

At the end, you may want to do a facial massage. With a small towel, wipe the excess oil off your hands. Look into your lover's eyes for a moment and acknowledge him. Place your hands as gently as possible on his face, cupping his face in your hands. Stroke his skin as lovingly as you possibly can. Softly pass by his eyelids, lips, forehead, and hair. Caress his cheeks and temples. Do it as if you were worshiping him. (You can also add a sexual massage.)

Electrifying Touch

When it comes to exploring new areas in our lovemaking techniques, we tend to go for the hot, strong, overt qualities instead of moving into the realm of the soft and sensuous. Slowing down and investigating every inch of your partner's skin can, on first investigation, seem too obvious.

But ask yourself: How often have I actually taken the time to discover my partner's erogenous zones? Have I asked her what she likes? When we begin to open up to our partners in these new, subtle ways, we open new doors to a fuller range of intimacy and connecting.

ESSENTIAL

Make a list of all the areas on your body that you either like to be touched or think that you might like to be touched. Then, list the five main places on your body that are your personal favorite erogenous zones. Share your lists with each other.

Erotic touch is an area that has a lot to explore—there are many esoteric ways of touching with hands, feet, and other body parts. For instance, Charles and Caroline Muir of Source Tantra teach a technique that refers to the penis as a wand or paintbrush that "paints" and strokes the outside of the vagina. In this form of foreplay, the man uses his penis, which is generally softly erect, to stroke the outer labia. As he gets the go-ahead signal from his partner, he comes closer to the vaginal opening, and strokes from clitoris to anus.

Here are a few more ideas on how to use touch in your foreplay:

- **Touch as light as a feather.** Touch as though you are stroking only the hair on the body. Use the fingertips, your palms, the back of your hand, or your cheek.
- **Light scratching.** If you have fingernails, try scratching your partner around his inner thighs, scrotum, buttocks, back, and head. Move slowly.
- **Light biting.** Nibbling on your partner may be very erotic. Try it around the ears and neck.
- **Pulling.** Gently but firmly pull the hair around your partner's genitals. Do this in a large handful, not little pieces.
- **Blowing.** Use your breath to blow on your partner—behind the ears, over the face, and over the genitals.

The Art of Kissing

Kissing is an art and can be enhanced with practice and intention. Our lips are extremely sensitive and receptive to stimulation. Many people hold their lips stiffly, not letting them relax and be open to the receiving and giving required for good kissing. Practice using your lips in a soft, open way. Part them slightly and keep them moist. This will heighten their sensitivity.

Practice pouting softly when you are by yourself. This relaxes the lips and exposes more of the fleshy interior. In general, become more aware of your lips. Try eating your meals more slowly than usual and really feel the food passing between your lips. Practice sucking on soft fruit, like a piece of mango, for the effect it has on your mouth and lips.

Kissing Techniques

When you are about to kiss, lick your lips to wet them, open your mouth a little, tip your head very slightly, and go softly forward. At first, leave your tongue out of it. Use your lips to gently explore the interior of your partner's lips. Move very slowly, but with confidence. Go deeper and open your mouth a bit more as you feel yourself going into the kiss. Create a slight amount of suction as you expand and open your mouth a little bigger.

Have a love contest to see how many different ways you can kiss. Challenge your lover to dueling lips and see how many different techniques you can come up with.

Take your lover's whole mouth into yours. Do this lovingly, as if you were exploring it for the first time. Eat them up—but gently. Now, if you wish to, you can do some "French" kissing—probing with your tongue into your lover's mouth and letting your lover do the same. Let your tongue slowly investigate rather than force its way into your partner's mouth. Tease and let yourself be teased. The subtler you are, the better. Kissing can go on for a long time if it's treated as a playful and erotic activity.

Music to My Ears

The ear is one of your main erogenous zones; it has many nerve endings, and it is situated near the neck, another highly erotic area. Ears are the gateway to hearing, one of the five senses. You can nurture your ears with music, a direct path to the soul.

The ear should be approached slowly, with a little teasing. Try a soft breath to start. Get close to the ear that is about to enjoy being the object of arousal. With slightly open lips, spread your warm breath around the ear and behind it. Move in with very soft and light kisses to the top area and the immediate hairline just above the ear. You might take a small piece of hair in your lips and give it a little pull, just to entice.

ESSENTIAL

Experience lovemaking as a dance, with many moves and sentiments that can be explored on the dance floor of the bedroom. Remember that whatever you are practicing in your lovemaking, the giver should be experiencing as much pleasure as the receiver.

Move down the ear slowly to the fleshier areas and the lobe. Kiss and gently blow. Speak to your partner with barely audible words, teasing a little if you want to, or reminding your partner to relax and breathe. As your partner begins to react by moving and making sounds, begin to press your lips a little harder and with more ardor. Take the lobe and lightly press and suck on it with your lips.

Love Bites

Move briefly to the neck just below the ear and place a few kisses there before moving back to the lobe. Now try a few light bites on the lower, fleshy part of the ear. Be gentle and playful. This is a bite to entice and show your passion; it is not meant to hurt.

After the bites, don't move away without first kissing and sucking a little more. You don't ever want to move away after a tease like a soft bite. Come back and treat the ear to a soft and sensual experience again before going on.

Talking Dirty

Even a little bit of naughty whispering can heat things up in the bedroom. Let's face it, nobody enjoys making love in total silence. Most people equate a more vocal partner with a more turned-on one. Virtually everyone finds sexy talk to be a turn-on (even if they didn't think they would). The key is to find the type and level of sex talk that you and your partner find the most exciting. This is tricky at first, because what you find sexy your partner might find obscene—or worse, disturbing. So proceed slowly, feeling out your partner's comfort level. If the two of you have previously been fairly quiet in bed, start out with a few louder-than-normal moans and some basic exclamations (Yes! More!). Gradually move on to more daring language, making sure to stay alert for any negative reactions from your partner.

ALERT

Many people are hesitant to use salty or X-rated language, even in the privacy of their own bedroom. This is where you need to provide a reminder that what happens in the bedroom stays in the bedroom. Nobody else will ever know that you or your partner used profanities in the privacy of your private space, so feel free to let the shocking words fly.

An Exercise in Sexual Communication

This exercise is both sensually fun and a good learning experience. It should be done with a partner, and you should expect to devote one hour for each person. Keep it light and see what you can discover about your partner and yourself.

This is a practice in sensual touch and will be accompanied by a simple but powerful communication technique. Essentially, you will be asking for different kinds of touch. This will be a practice in learning what you like, how to ask for it, and training your partner in what you want.

This is an activity you can come back to more than once; each time, you can be more detailed and precise. Practicing clear communication in this fun way will help in those times when it's more difficult to communicate.

Feeling worthy of asking for intimacy and having someone honor that request is difficult for many of us. But what you discover is that when you do bring a little more humility and vulnerability into your life, your partner will see more beauty in you than ever before. When you reveal yourself in new ways, you are saying, "I trust you, and I am entrusting my most vulnerable self to you." That kind of thing is irresistible—even if it is a bit new and awkward. Think of awkwardness as a sign of innocence, a signal that you and your lover are entering uncharted territory together. This is the kind of thing that keeps love alive and fresh.

Let's Begin

To begin the exercise, set the scene by lighting a few strategically placed candles. Scent the room, decorate it with flowers, and have massage oil and something to drink ready for your use. Make sure the room is warm. When you're ready, proceed as follows:

1. **Make a positive statement about the touch you are currently receiving.** Keep it simple. "I love the way you look at me when you touch me." Or, "I love the way your fingertips feel on my face."
2. **Ask for a change.** Keep this simple, too. "Would you please use a little more pressure?" Or, "Would you try that a little faster to see how it feels?"
3. **When your partner responds, give thanks:** "Mmmm . . . that's great." Anything in a positive tone will do. That doesn't mean you necessarily liked the change. It is okay to say: "Wow. I thought I'd like that, but I was wrong. Thank you for helping me learn that about myself."

Difficulties in Communication

If your partner seems reluctant to communicate, use positive messages to encourage speaking. Ask a multiple-choice question such as, "Would you like me to do this a little harder or softer?" If you're the one who is shier about speaking up, try to find the courage to ask for your partner's encouragement. You might say, for example, "Do you really want to hear what I like? If you do, I'd like you to remind me of that now and then."

Here are some questions to see how you did with this exercise:

- How did this experience make you feel?
- What did you notice about your breathing?
- Were you able to take the focused time that your lover offered and enjoy it?

- Was it hard to receive that much time and energy from your lover?
- Did you get nervous and want to "give back" before your receiving time was over?

Each time you practice this exercise, check back with these questions to see if your responses have changed.

CHAPTER 10

Assume the Position

New positions are possibly the best way to introduce variety and interest into a sexual relationship. They can be exciting, a little challenging, and often inspiring. There are really only a handful of basic positions, but there are many, many variations on each of the basic ones, and practicing variety will help any couple reach greater pleasure.

Yin and Yang

Many Eastern cultures believe that male and female energies run opposite to each other. The Taoists say that man pulls his sexual and life energy (yang) from his feet, up through his penis and then upward into his heart. Woman, on the other hand, takes her energy (yin) from the top, down through her heart and then to her genitals. Hence, the war of the sexes—she needs a heart connection before she has sex; he needs sex before he can have a heart connection. How do they proceed?

Your choice of positions can have a major influence on your yin/yang relationship. Yin is the receptive principle. Yang is the active principle. The position you choose, and its appropriateness for your particular needs, can make the difference in whether you experience a female/male energy dance or a war of the sexes.

When a woman opens up her sexual repertoire to include trying positions where she is on top and in control, she becomes the "male" principle or the yang in the sex act at that moment. This empowers her and can give her a growing confidence in taking a more sexually active role. When the male is on the bottom, he can move into his feminine yin side. This takes the heat off, so to speak. He can relax. He doesn't have to be in charge and perform. The simple act of trying a new position can often be transformative for a relationship.

There's Always Something New

Even the most experienced and mature lovers can always discover a new sexual move, technique, or position. This can be exciting, even if you currently enjoy a satisfying sex life. When you investigate a new position, you can count on having new things to talk about and learn together. Exploring new positions should be fun, and you should be prepared to communicate with your partner and laugh at yourself if you don't quite get it right away. You'll probably find that some positions will work well for you and some just won't at all.

The more positions you try out, the more your awkwardness or reluctance will disappear and the easier it will become to learn new ones. You'll find yourself becoming willing to try other new things with your lover. That's what makes exploring different positions so important. This form of trying something new will often lead to a transformed sexual relationship. For couples who want to learn and add to their sexual repertoire, exploring new positions can be one of the best ways to do it.

The Perfect Fit

Experimenting with different positions may also help solve the problem of the imperfect fit. That is, a woman with a large vagina may end up with a man who has a smaller penis. Or, on the contrary, a woman with a tight vagina may have a lover whose penis is too big for her, causing her pain during intercourse.

A couple that experiences these types of problems has to try new positions to get the very best out of their lovemaking. Positions that hurt the woman or don't allow her to move her hips and adjust her body to her partner's are going to contribute to an uncomfortable sexual experience.

If the woman or man can't communicate problems like this, the couple may begin to shy away from sexual activity. This can be the beginning of a downhill swing in the relationship. The couple may never come out of it, all because neither person could say they weren't comfortable with the way their sexual experiences were going. Exploring new positions can help.

The vagina will, in most cases, expand or tighten to fit the penis. Foreplay for the woman makes a tremendous amount of difference. It's a rare case that the fit just won't work.

A Great Variety of Positions

There are as many positions as there are possibilities in the creative mind. When trying them out, keep the communication going. Tell your partner what you like and what doesn't work for you.

Very few of us are mind readers, so when in doubt, ask. If your partner is quieter than you are, encourage him to speak up. Ask multiple choice questions:

- Do you prefer that I do this faster or slower?
- Do you like this harder or softer?
- Should we move on to another position or would you like me to continue?

Even if the answer is "none of the above," just knowing that you care can give your partner the courage to speak up. Remember, you both really want to know what the other one wants and likes.

There's More Than One Way

There are many subtle variations on each major group of positions. If a new position isn't working for you, don't abandon it right away. Try moving a leg to the left or right, or put a pillow under yourself to lift your pelvis, or shift from one knee to the other.

Have pillows of varying sizes and shapes like crescent moons, rounds, and squares available to use under your head, arms, legs, buttocks, tummy, and feet to subtly change angles and positions. Don't be afraid to get creative!

The Missionary Position

The missionary position is probably one of the most widely used positions during sex. In this position, the woman lies on her back with her legs bent and her knees pointing up with her feet on the bed. Her partner lies on top of her, generally with his knees on the bed or other surface. The man supports himself with his arms, and the woman's hips support his hips.

The man does the thrusting and most of the movement in this position. It's a somewhat difficult position for the woman to move freely, especially if the man is larger than she is and leans on her during lovemaking.

Basic variations of the missionary position include having the woman wrap her legs over the ankles, thighs, or buttocks of her partner. She can even move them up to his waist and back. These variations sometimes happen spontaneously as the woman get more excited and turned on. The natural reaction is to move closer to create more contact as the lovemaking progresses.

These positions can stimulate the G-spot and the interior vaginal spots that women identify as pleasure producing. They are also great for eye contact, whispers, loving words, and kissing; and the partners can put their arms around each other. Traditional thrusting, however, doesn't do much for most women because there's no clitoral stimulation.

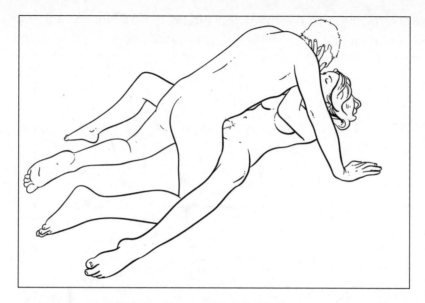

The missionary position is perhaps the most widely used sexual position.

The Coital Alignment Technique

Also known as CAT, the coital alignment technique is a modified frontal position that improves the woman's stimulation. The CAT is similar to the missionary position, except that the man rises up and moves about four inches forward (up her body). In this position, he can use a combination of small thrusts and rubbing his body up and down to get the woman more excited.

The rubbing action, which both partners can do in rhythm with each other, rubs the man's pubic bone on the woman's pubic bone and clitoral hood. This friction adds enough contact with the clitoris to have her reach orgasm in the act of intercourse. Generally, the CAT position has partners very close, with arms around each other, so that they can create the traction to get the up-and-down rhythm going. It's this back-and-forth friction that excites the woman and may make the man last longer, too.

The Yawning Position

Vulnerable and erotic, this position could become one of your favorites. The woman lies on her back and places her legs up and over the shoulders of her partner, who is on top of her. The legs can rest on his shoulders with very little strain to the man. She should not use much of a pillow, if any, under her buttocks, as this will limit her mobility.

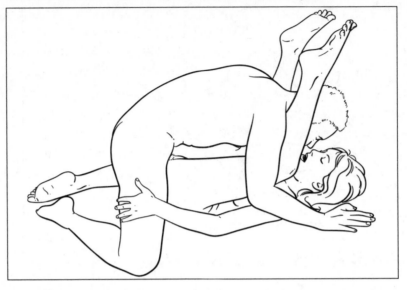

The yawning position lets the woman rest her legs on the man's shoulders.

With the man on top, you can go from the missionary position to the yawning position very easily. Thrusting should begin gently, as this is a vulnerable position for some women. With her legs on his shoulders, she will have the leverage to lift her pelvis easily and affect the angle of penetration.

ESSENTIAL

Most women eventually begin to have orgasms at some point in their lives, but not necessarily every time they have intercourse. More women experience clitoral orgasms as opposed to vaginal or G-spot orgasms.

One of the benefits of this position is that the woman can easily rotate her hips for maximum contact to her G-spot. The rotating also stimulates the man and they can both control the movement and the thrusting easily and freely. In this posture the hands are free to stimulate other erogenous zones. The man can use his hands and fingers on the clitoris, breasts, face or any other area on the woman's body where he knows her pleasure will be enhanced. The woman's hands are free to caress her partner's face, back, neck, thighs, legs, and scrotum.

She can assist him in having an orgasm but not ejaculating in this position because she can read his energy easily. She is able to move, do her Kegels to grip him firmly, or lie still so he won't orgasm too soon. Lying still, in a heightened state of arousal, with the woman squeezing her PC muscles in this position is pure ecstasy. This is a good way to let the man come back to a more stable state if he is feeling that he might be getting close to ejaculating. Lie still and, if appropriate, pump your PC muscles slowly and keep him just at the edge of excitement.

A variation on this position calls for the woman to straighten her legs and firmly push the backs of her legs away from the man, so that her feet move closer to her head. In doing so she puts a greater angle on her pelvis, and consequently the man's penis accesses the G-spot better. She is more in control of the thrusting in this variation and can control the deep versus shallow thrusts and the speed of the thrusting. This is a little more difficult for some women, but try it before you decide that it's not for you. The more of an angle you are able to put on the vagina and penis, the more pressure will be applied, causing greater pleasure.

Splitting a Bamboo Position

Sir Richard Burton's translation of the *Kama Sutra* includes the following passage: "When the woman places one of her legs on her lover's shoulder, and stretches the other out, and then places the latter on his shoulder, and stretches the other out, it is called the *splitting of a bamboo.*"

In this position, the woman lies on her back and can be propped up by pillows placed at her back. Her partner squats, kneels, or sits on his feet with a slightly forward tilt. The woman has one leg bent with her foot on the floor or bed. The other leg is on the man's shoulder, with the ankle hooked on it or straight up in the air and held by her partner's hand. At the couple's own pace, the legs are then placed in the opposite position. As in the *Kama Sutra* description, the legs are at one moment split one way and then the other way.

This is a wonderful position for making the subtle shifts that are often required for effective G-spot stimulation. The woman can grind and rotate her hips or undulate and use her PC muscles to create greater pleasure for both herself and her partner. The up-and-down motion of the legs creates an arc that rubs, like the motion of a windshield wiper, back and forth across the G-spot area. This position is more advanced than others, but give it a try. You may surprise yourself.

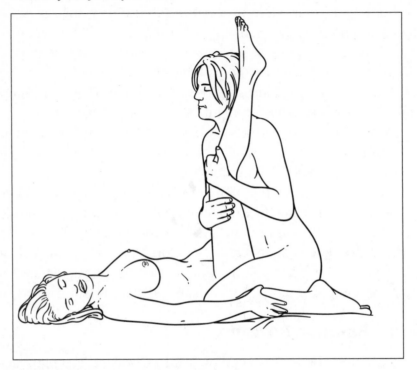

The "splitting the bamboo" sex position.

Woman on Top

Empowering, satisfying, vulnerable, creative, and edgy—all these adjectives and more can be applied to positions where the woman is on top. Often portrayed as either goddess or slut, a woman may have a difficult time assuming both manifestations in one body. Sometimes women want to be controlled and sometimes they want to be the one in charge. Assuming the top position can have the effect of bringing out the powerful animal passion in any woman. Men will get more of what they want with such a multiflavored lover.

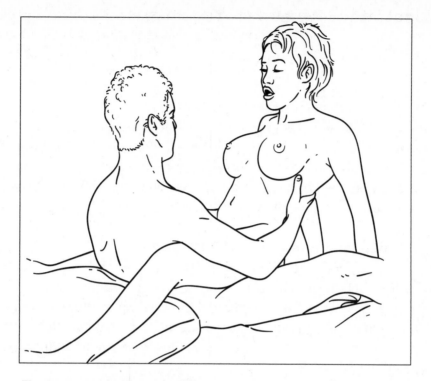

The "woman on top" sex position.

It's a wonderful lover who will allow the woman her full repertoire of sexual expression. However, women themselves collude with social mores by holding back their sexual energy. It's difficult to overcome the training that the family, community, religion, and culture have put us through. Personal fears often keep women from exploring a fuller range of possibilities when it comes to sexuality. If you haven't tried any of the many top positions, now is the time to try. Be gentle with yourself, and be sure to tell your partner of any vulnerable feelings you are experiencing.

As the lovemaking progresses, you can move through each one of these variations one by one, like a dance. You can perfect this dance by staying aware and limber. Take the lead sometimes, and let your partner lead at other times. Remember to use your hands liberally to caress your partner. The more loving your touch, the more total the experience.

Variations of the Woman on Top Position

The basic configuration for the range of woman on top positions is for the man to be lying on his back and the woman to straddle him, but there are many variations to this basic position—for instance, the woman can be facing forward, sideways, or backward. The majority of these positions call for the woman to be facing forward so that there's eye contact, and the couple may kiss and speak to each other. The forward types are also the best for G-spot stimulation. With the woman on top, the man can have his legs flat along the bed or bent, with knees pointing up. The woman can experiment with any of the following variations:

Fluttering and Soaring Butterfly

This position, described in the *Kama Sutra*, is performed with the woman's feet on the bed. This allows the woman to raise and lower herself onto the man. The woman is in control of the rhythm, depth of thrusting, speed, and angle of penetration. It takes strong thighs to maintain this position for a length of time. The man can use his hands to help support the woman and guide her timing.

Woman Upright, with Knees on the Bed

This modification of the butterfly position offers a great range of motion because the woman can move up and down as well as forward and backward. She is closer to her partner's face and is often supporting herself with one or both hands. It is possible for her to use one of her hands to caress her lover's face and body.

FACT

Remember that even if a new position looks like a lot of fun, what really matters is how it feels to you and your partner. Be sure to communicate throughout the entire process. You can always adjust a position based on how you and your partner feel about it.

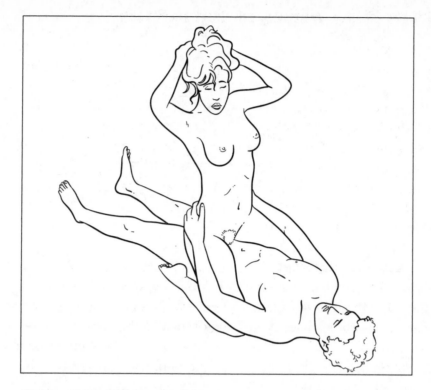

Woman on top, with knees on bed.

Both Legs Straight Out in Front

This position is a little more challenging. The woman will have to use her hands to support herself while moving up and down. Try sliding back and forth on your man, but be careful not to hurt him, especially if you are average to large in body size. Try this one facing away from your man, too.

Leaning Down over the Man's Chest, with Knees on the Bed

This particular position is a good one for clitoral stimulation because the two of you can rub against each other, as in the CAT position. The woman can guide her lover to apply maximum friction where she needs it most.

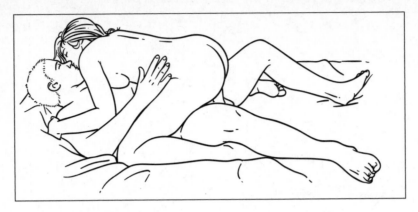

Woman on top, leaning on man.

Alternating Feet

In this position, the woman has one leg with the foot on the bed and the other leg with the knee on the bed. This is a good option for women who prefer stimulation of one side of their vagina or G-spot over the other. It's also very powerful for the woman to put her hand under the man's buttocks on the side with the foot on the bed. She can gently pull him closer and rock him back and forth

Lying on Top

In this position, the woman lies on top of the man, moving up and down in order to stimulate her clitoris.

Reverse Cowgirl

In this position, the woman sits on top of the man, with her back to him. This allows the woman a wide range of movement.

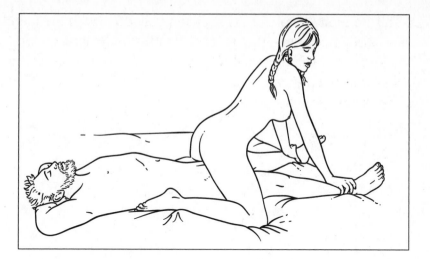

The reverse cowgirl position.

Rear-Entry Positions

Without a doubt, rear-entry positions are some of the best positions—they enhance G-spot stimulation, they have the advantage of leaving the man's hands free to caress and fondle the breasts, and variety is easy to come by. With rear-entry positions, you can adjust the angle and depth of penetration and the ways you move. This allows the woman to adapt the experience for herself while having a lot of room to increase the pleasure for her partner. It also enables the woman or the man to stimulate her clitoris. For some women, this is an important part of intercourse.

ALERT

Rear-entry positions aren't always the most appropriate; the moment must be right. Sometimes it's just more appropriate to be facing each other. Eye contact, breath connection, heart connection, and intimacy are all facilitated through facing your partner.

Men may find that they are turned on by the increased control in these positions. You can be in control of the depth, speed, and rhythm. You have a wonderful, archetypal view of your partner, reminiscent of ancient or primitive man. Men can feel powerful and still maintain sensitivity with their partner.

This position is probably most commonly done with the man kneeling behind the woman, with the upper half of his body upright. Some couples also like to do a variation in which the man leans forward so he is on all fours as well, but this can be uncomfortable or tricky, especially if there's a big size difference in the partners.

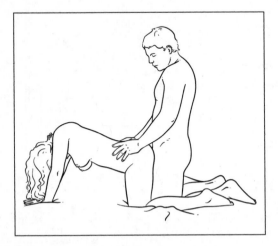

The rear entry (or "doggie style") position.

Try a Few Variations

Try having the woman lean forward and lay her head down. This is a good position for stimulating the man by caressing his scrotum or his inner thighs. You can also help him stay focused on nonejaculatory pleasure by cupping his scrotum in your hands and gently applying pressure with a downward pull.

Be gentle and always ask first if it's something he would like you to try. You may also wish to apply pressure to his perineum (the external area between the anus and the scrotum that covers his prostate gland, or the male G-spot). This will help keep him from going over the top, so to speak.

Another variation of the rear-entry position is one where both partners are lying flat on their stomachs, with the man on top of the woman. This can feel suffocating for the woman—indeed, it allows for very little range of movement—but it can sometimes be a good strategy for taking a breather or slowing things down to prolong orgasm.

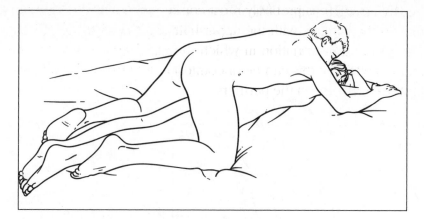

Rear entry, with man lying flat on top of woman.

Yab-Yum Positions

The basic yab-yum position is a little-known but excellent position to explore. Lovers are face-to-face and heart-to-heart. They are able to keep eye contact, kiss, and caress each other. This position is the best one for extending the sexual experience because it prevents the man from thrusting so much that he ejaculates too quickly. It allows for the deep connection that makes the extended lovemaking experience magical.

In this position, the man sits cross-legged on the bed or floor and the woman sits astride him. She is facing him and has her legs wrapped around him, with the soles of her feet coming together behind him. Both partners have their arms wrapped around each other, and their faces are very close. The woman can put a firm pillow under her buttocks to help with the pressure on her lover's thighs, if necessary.

If you're not very comfortable in the basic yab-yum position, you may modify it as follows: The man can sit on the edge of the bed or a padded hassock (footstool) with his legs on the floor while the woman sits facing him on his lap. Make sure the man's legs are parallel to the floor from the knees to the hip. This is a good modification for people with lower back problems.

The yab-yum is a great position to use when the man starts getting too close to ejaculation. It's a position that is easy for the man to stay aroused in even when there is a minimum of movement. By combining fast, hot movements with slow, steady rocking and even stillness, you can create a dance. This allows you to remain in a high state of ecstatic connection for virtually as long as you want. It's a little more daring and advanced, but it's well worth it.

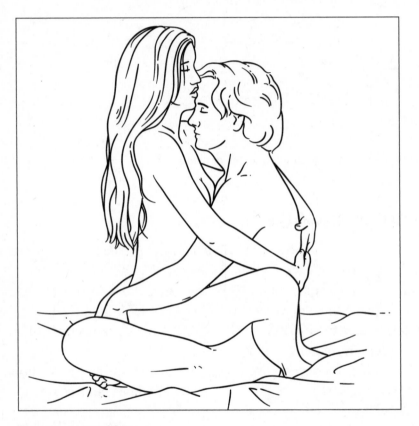

The yab yum position.

Clasping Positions

The clasping positions are postures in which the woman and the man maintain a straight-legged, rather rigid posture in respect to each other. Clasping comes from the idea that the woman must clasp or hold on to the man's penis with her vaginal muscles and thighs. These positions don't allow for much movement. When the legs are stiff, the feet can't be employed to help lift the pelvic region, so it's hard to accomplish any sort of rhythmic swinging motion of the hips.

You can try any of the following clasping positions:

- Woman on her back, with the man on top
- Man on his back, with the woman on top
- Woman on her stomach, with the man on top
- Side by side and facing toward each other or in a spooning position

The clasping positions have an advantage in situations where the man has a large penis and the woman has a smallish vagina. It can be very uncomfortable and possibly dangerous for a woman in this situation to completely accept hard, deep thrusting from her partner. Because the closed legs prevent the penis from deep penetration but give ample friction to the man, these positions can facilitate the love act. On the other hand, a woman with a generous vagina partnered with a man with a smaller penis won't get as much out of these positions.

The advantage of any position that allows for shallower rather than deeper penetration is that the woman's G-spot will get more action, as may her clitoris. Remember that the G-spot is nearer the entrance of the vagina, rather than back near the cervix. When there is more frequent thrusting and the man's penetration is shallower, the head of the penis contacts the woman's G-spot a greater percentage of the time, so she'll get excited more quickly.

Spooning Positions

Spooning positions are a wonderful addition to any couple's repertoire of lovemaking. Greatly nurturing, they are especially appropriate for either the very beginning or the very end of a lovemaking session. Partners can use spooning positions to connect deeply before making love or they can use them at the very end, for holding and lying still in those magical moments before drifting off to sleep.

These positions can be used whether the man has an erect penis or not. Just holding each other in these positions has its place in any lovemaking situation. They can also be used when the two of you desire to make love but the woman is low on energy or both of you are more tired than usual and you want to stay very mellow. With the woman in front and the man behind holding her, the couple can gently undulate, whether they are having intercourse or just bonding.

ALERT

When trying any new position, take it slowly at first and stay very conscious of your partner and his feelings. New positions can trigger long-buried emotions and feelings of vulnerability. Keep the communication open and be willing to stop and explore the feelings that are coming up for both of you.

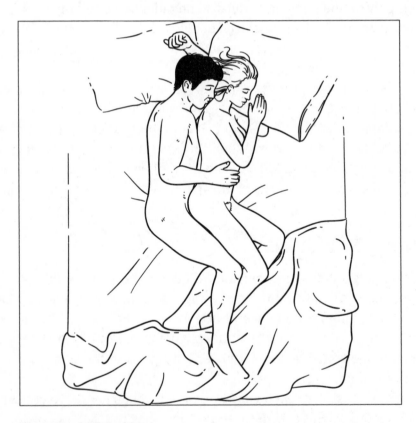

The "spooning" position.

Generally, you assume a position similar to spoons lying next to each other. Lie front to front or back to front, with either the man or the woman in front, depending on who needs the most cuddling. Bring the arm and hand that is under you to the front, under the person in front, so that you can hold them near their heart area. The other hand can come over the top to hold their pelvic region close to yours. Pull them to you and snuggle up close.

Many couples start out with the spooning position and then have one partner move into other positions to up the excitement level. Try going into the T-shaped position. The man remains lying on his side, as with spooning, while the woman gets on her back and slides around until she is perpendicular to him, so her hips meet his and her legs are draped over his body (her feet are usually planted behind him on the bed to allow her some leverage for movement). This position allows for new and unique sensations, due to the angle of penetration, and it also provides a good angle for clitoral stimulation by either the man or woman.

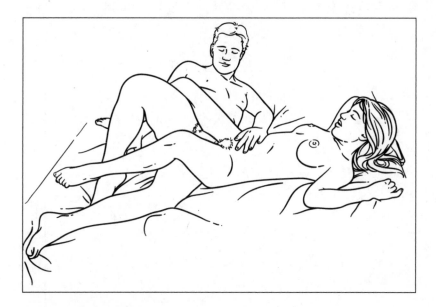

The "T-shaped" position.

Advanced Positions

If you feel like you've mastered all the routine positions or just feel the urge to expand your horizons, you might want to try a move advanced position.

Here are a few types of advanced positions you can try:

Standing Positions

This can be a little tricky if there's a height difference—in which case, the man might want to lift the woman while she wraps her legs around him. To make things easier, she can sit on a counter or piece of furniture, or lean back against a wall. To make things even more challenging, try an arrangement where the man is standing while the woman is upside-down, with her head near the floor (she can support herself by placing her hands on the floor).

Sitting Positions

This may or may not be challenging, depending on which variation you choose. The woman is usually sitting in the man's lap, but she can face either toward or away from the man. Adjust the sensations by having the woman lean as far backward or forward as she can manage.

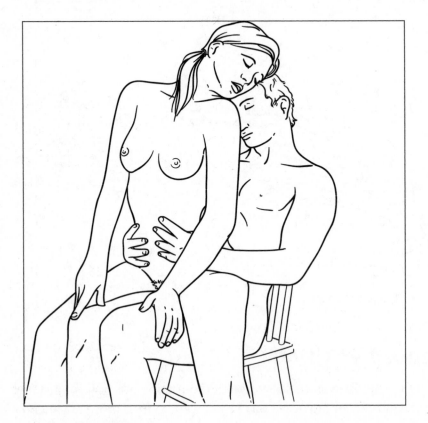

A sitting sex position.

Acrobatic Positions

These are the type of positions that generally require considerable flexibility and/or creativity. They would include arrangements in which one or both partners are upside-down or lying diagonally across the bed, or where one partner is balanced precariously on a single limb or appendage (either their own or their partner's).

Try these positions slowly, proceeding with caution. Some of them are risky and can cause injury, especially if you aren't very flexible or have any type of physical limitation (such as a bad back).

Positions for Conceiving

Over the course of history, couples have managed to conceive via just about every sexual position you can imagine. But if you really want to get pregnant—especially if you've been trying for a while with no luck—you might want to focus your efforts on specific positions.

ALERT

As you probably already know, timing is critical to conceiving. Most people believe this is what you should concentrate on, as opposed to your choice of positions. The most important thing isn't how you have sex, but when. Track your menstrual cycle to pinpoint your most fertile days, and try using an ovulation test to find out when you are most likely to conceive.

Many people believe the missionary position is best for conception, especially if the woman lies in place (perhaps even lying with her legs raised) for a few minutes following sex. Others believe the rear-entry positions are best because they allow for deeper penetration.

There is no scientific evidence to prove that one position is more likely to help you conceive, but it couldn't hurt to try. Spend one month primarily having sex in one position and see what happens. If that doesn't work, try a new position the next month.

Positions for Pregnant Women

Many women are surprised to find that they have an increase in sexual desire when pregnant, especially during the first few months. This is probably due to the increase in hormones, or simply the fact that they are basking in that pregnancy glow. At the same time, many men find that their wives suddenly seem hotter and sexier when pregnant (those swollen and enlarged breasts surely don't hurt matters!). Bottom line: This is the perfect recipe for some really hot sex. Bonus: There are no contraception-related worries or interruptions to spoil the mood.

The good news: Barring any medical conditions or special circumstances, most sex positions are perfectly safe for pregnant women. It's probably a good idea to skip the really challenging moves that require her to contort her body, but other than that, you can go wild. Toward the end of the pregnancy, you might need to make a few minor adjustments, such as avoiding positions in which the man's weight is on the woman's belly. Let the woman's comfort level be the guide. Needless to say, you should immediately stop if the woman feels the slightest bit of discomfort.

ALERT

Sex—and, more specifically, orgasms—can often seem to trigger labor. So if a woman is past her due date and eager to have her baby, it might be time for her and her partner to hit the sheets.

Never Stop Exploring

There are many other erotic positions to explore. See if you can discover some for yourselves. Just to give you an idea, there's one called the twinning branches. To get an idea of how this position works, open up both of your hands, make the scissors shape with your first and second fingers on each hand and put them together to "cut" each other. The resulting shape is the position that the two of you would assume. This position is comfortable and is good for relaxing and resting while making love. Women will find that one side or the other may feel better. See which side suits you.

You'll be able to explore some more exotic ideas and variations in Chapter 14, so have fun and keep in mind that you are taking each other on an erotic journey. Draw your partner in by keeping close contact with soft, intimate eyes. Study each other's facial expressions. Stay very connected. Breathe deeply.

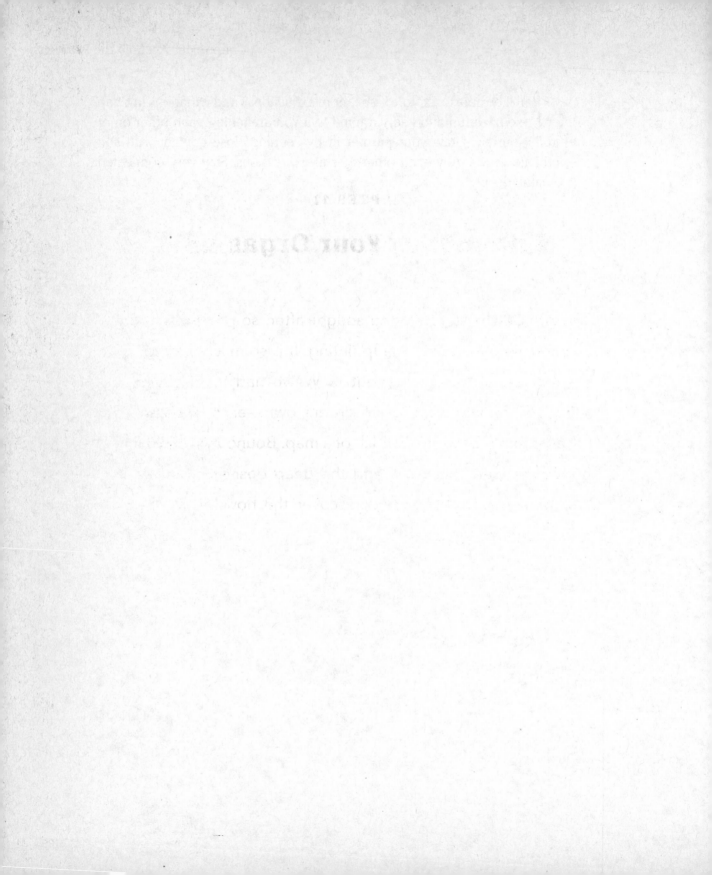

CHAPTER 11

Enhancing Your Orgasms

The big O—so exquisite, so sought after, so powerful, or so soon, so elusive, so disappointing. It is so much and yet we really know so little about it. We've had to discover the world of sex and orgasm on our own—each of us an intrepid explorer without much of a map. Bound by instinct, hormones, peer pressure, and the deep desire to please and be pleased, we seek to discover the how-tos of the great, soul-fulfilling orgasm.

Why Do Humans Experience Orgasms?

You might wonder why people have orgasms—not that anyone's complaining, mind you. But orgasms are, when you think about it, kind of a luxury. Humans can reproduce—and perhaps even have a fairly satisfying sex life—without having an orgasm. So what's the purpose? The most basic answer to the question of why humans have orgasms is procreation.

It's true that humans can conceive without orgasms. But it's not a matter of necessity. It's more of an incentive. To ensure that humans will continue to reproduce, nature has given us the orgasm as a sensual reward. Why would we have the drive to have sexual relations if there wasn't something very enjoyable about the act? After all, the clitoris has no biological function other than pleasure, and yet it has the highest concentration of nerve endings in the whole body.

FACT

Scientists have discovered that when a woman experiences an orgasm, her cervix actually dips down during each contraction and "sips" the semen up into the uterus. It's perfectly clear that throughout evolutionary history both men and women needed orgasmic pleasure to drive the survival of the species.

While no two orgasms are ever really alike, nor are we able to describe each man's or woman's individual experience, we know the basic path the orgasm takes each time we are graced with the experience. The important part is that the orgasm depends on each person's capacity to feel and receive pleasure.

Pleasure Is Your Birthright

Nature has given us the sex organs, the hormones, and the desire to have sex. We have the capacity to fantasize, to think about sex, and to actualize the act through lovemaking. It is your birthright to have the fullest sexual pleasure you can possibly experience. You may choose to fully partake of your sexual potential, or you may choose to abstain. And, of course, you may choose anything in between.

You, and only you, are responsible for how much pleasure you experience. Your partner is not the responsible one. If you hold ideas about the "shoulds" and "shouldn'ts" of sex that limit your capacity for pleasure, it's time to ferret them out. In a sense, the mind can be the greatest sex organ or the worst inhibitor of bodily pleasure.

If you're openly curious about your own sexual response cycle and give yourself permission to have pleasure, you will open up to new worlds. If you shut down your natural openness through false expectations and limiting beliefs, your capacity for pleasure diminishes. Taking charge of your sexual pleasure will empower you and free you in ways that extend beyond the bedroom.

Learn to Enjoy Yourself Again

Men and women are supposed to be good at sex, yet we live in a culture that hides sexuality or confuses it with symbols of power or powerlessness. A society like ours does not educate its young adults in how to honor and love their own bodies. With rare exceptions, every young person must either reinvent the wheel or overcome huge prejudices in order to learn about sexuality and sensuality.

Inability to experience orgasm is a frustrating problem that directly affects women's self-esteem and relationships. To add insult to injury, many men ejaculate before their partner is even warmed up! These obstacles can frustrate couples so much that they decide sex isn't worth it.

The Keys to Great Pleasure

Don't get stressed out by your quest to achieve the perfect orgasm. Trust that with love, practice, and playful innocence you can begin to have the kinds of sexual experiences you always dreamed of. The following list summarizes the basic ingredients for expanding the capacity to orgasm:

- Learn to relax. Take hot baths at quiet times. Take time for yourself. Go away for the weekend to a spa all by yourself.
- Become an excellent breather.
- Stay conscious during sex; don't drift away.

- Learn to meditate. It will help you learn to focus your attention.
- Know your body and what you like.
- Make noise. Sound helps your partner know what you like, and it helps you let go into a deeper experience.
- Do your Kegel exercises.

Notice that there isn't anything on this list that even hints at technique. While speed, timing, placement, and new techniques are wonderful, they won't help you focus and expand into the pleasure. Personal mastery over the domain of your mind and body will.

Staying Conscious and Aware

Eye gazing with your partner will put you in full awareness and bring you to the present with your lover. Leaving the lights on or lighting candles during sex and keeping your eyes open is the best way to bond with your partner. When we are fully available and open to being seen, our capacity for merging and orgasm goes way up. Once you get used to relating in this way, you won't want to go back to the dark.

Learn to Meditate

What does meditation have to do with great sex? It helps us learn to focus our attention. One of the main things that gets in the way of the orgasmic response in women is worrying. We can't get the kids, bills, phone calls, groceries, business, and so much more off our minds. Meditation for as little as twenty minutes three times a week will give you a wonderful new tool to draw on for relaxation and focus.

Do Your Kegel Exercises

It can't be emphasized enough—both men and women need to strengthen their PC muscles and use them! Once you're good at doing Kegels, you will actually be able to turn yourself on! You can do up to 200 at a time in just five to ten minutes, and it can be done anytime and anywhere—while you're driving, sitting at your desk, in a meeting . . . you get the picture.

Kegel exercises facilitate the flow of blood to your genitals and they keep your pelvic floor muscles healthy. If you do these twice a day, you will notice a difference. See Chapter 5 to review how Kegel exercises are done.

Unlearning Old Habits

It can be very difficult for some women to open their legs into wide positions. The vulnerability of exposing their genitals to be seen, touched, and honored can be a lot to handle. But if you bring a gentle will, a playful and loving heart, and a little patience to the practice, you can reap the benefits of expanding your orgasmic capabilities. Unlearning old habits is always hard but usually worth the work and focus.

Mastery of Your Breath

Breathing is not a conscious activity for most humans. We expect to just know how to do it. Yet the key to greater health and vitality, experiences of expanded consciousness, and the full-body orgasm is mastery of the breath. Yogis place a great emphasis on learning to deepen and lengthen the breath. Becoming conscious of the breath and its patterns is the first step in the process of expanding orgasm.

We're a culture of chest breathers. Chest breathing causes adrenaline secretions that can lead to panic and fear. We're taught to suck our stomachs in and wear tight belts and clothing. This pushes our breath into our chests. We don't know how to belly breathe.

ESSENTIAL

Discovering your G-spot and beginning to develop the capacity to have vaginal orgasms in addition to clitoral ones can have the outcome of opening you up. Remember to breathe deeply into your belly, be patient, and love yourself.

You can't relax your genitals when you're holding in your stomach. The body becomes rigid. It's very difficult to tighten and hold your genitals when your stomach is full of breath. Try it. A relaxed body leads to a more relaxed attitude, which will lead to a more relaxed life. The way in which you breathe can make a vast difference in the quality of your orgasms and your life.

Breathing Issues among Women

Women who don't orgasm easily often hold their breath as they get more turned on. As they approach a kind of transition stage on the way to peak arousal, say a seven or eight on a scale of ten, they will often hold their breath, and then nothing happens. The result is that the energy must be built up again, only to have the same thing happen repeatedly. It becomes difficult to transition smoothly to the next level of sensations.

As arousal gets going in women, they will often begin to breathe a little faster. If they become aware of their breath, they can then begin to "drive" the experience by purposely doing faster, focused breathing to increase blood flow and arousal. It helps, exactly as meditation does, to focus the energy and move from a sense of separateness to one of being merged with the energy.

Good Breathing for Men

Once they are practiced at awareness, men can, when they notice their breath getting faster, consciously breathe slower and more fully. This allows them to move the sexual excitement through their body instead of unconsciously going right past all those exquisite feelings and going over the top.

Making Noise

Breath and sound go hand in hand. Deep, resonant, low-register notes can transform your orgasmic abilities. They open up the body cavity because the mouth is usually pretty wide open and the energy flow gets much more accentuated. Sound and breath can lead to multiple orgasms.

Making noise during sexual play is a turn-on and helps us know where our partner is in the sexual response cycle. The signs of arousal and stimulation, especially in women, are very hard to interpret even with sound added. When we open up our mouths to let sound out, we literally open up the body cavity and allow the energy and pleasure to be transported through us.

It's almost physically impossible to make deep sounds while in orgasm and hold your pelvic region tight at the same time. Moaning opens up the pelvic region and relaxes the genital area, greatly enhancing the full-body orgasms that follow.

If making sounds is new for you, let your partner know that you'd like to try it. It can even feel a little silly at first, but being vulnerable will draw you and your partner closer, so go for it. Consciously bring sound to your love-making so you can really see how it works.

Positions for Increasing Orgasmic Response

Changing and varying positions can be very helpful in finding new ways to stimulate the G-spot in women. They are also valuable in helping men last longer and achieve mastery over their ejaculations. In addition, trying alternative positions keeps the energy new between partners and invites open exploration.

Positions that enhance the connection between the G-spot and the penis in coitus are ones that place the angle of penetration such that the head of the penis is pointing to the top wall of the vagina. Positions in which the woman is on her back and has her legs up or on her partner's shoulders work well to achieve this angle.

When the woman is on top, she can help guide the penis in the right direction and to the right depth for maximum effect. Positions that directly affect the clitoris are the missionary and its close cousin, the CAT. It's best to rub back and forth in these positions rather than just thrusting in and out. Thrusting, in general, pulls on the labia minora and the clitoral hood, but the stimulation is, at best, indirect.

Men, Make It Easier on Yourselves

Unfortunately, the positions that create the most friction for women do so for men as well. If you are having problems with ejaculating faster than you'd like to, you may have to train yourself to last longer. Men, if your partner has already had a clitoral orgasm before you have intercourse and you aren't yet able to last as long as you'd like, try positions that don't cause the most fric-tion. Those would be the missionary position, spooning, certain positions that use furniture, sex while standing, and any position where the two of you can eye gaze and stay in deep communication.

Thrusting Patterns

Great lovers have learned that sex isn't just about in and out. Men, when you're doing most of the movement, spend some time teasing by staying shallow and then surprising your partner with three deep thrusts. Create a dance of churning, deep thrusting, and then shallow thrusting, and then reverse the order.

A classic pattern of thrusting, suggested by one of the ancient erotic books, is nine deep thrusts, then one shallow (and slow); eight deep thrusts, then two shallow; seven deep thrusts, then three shallow; and so on. Go slowly, eye gaze, and take deep breaths into your bellies. The breath carries the intense feelings throughout your body. It translates the acceptance of the pleasure to your brain. This thrusting pattern allows the man to get very excited and then transfer that excitement to the woman.

Shallow thrusting stimulates the G-spot area more effectively. Generally, a woman will like deep thrusting and shallow thrusting at different times during arousal. Ask your partner what she likes best. Try making up your own patterns with the help of your partner.

Ejaculatory Mastery for Men

This is one of the most common complaints and frustrations men have about sex: "How can I stop from having quick orgasms? Sometimes I ejaculate after fifteen seconds! My partner is not able to climax. Please help me."

What's the rush? The fast ejaculation may be the result of guilty feelings, fear of getting caught while masturbating, being out of touch with one's own body, or honesty and trust issues with one's partners. As a result, men have very often trained themselves to come too quickly.

Over thousands of years, the tantrics and Taoists have developed simple, easy, and fun techniques to help men train themselves to last longer. While whole books are written on this subject, a good grasp of the essence of the practices can be given here. All you need is training, intention, focused attention, and practice. If you put in some effort, the result will be well worth it. Most men see significant results in just two weeks of practice.

ESSENTIAL

Ejaculation mastery is the first step toward multiple orgasms for men. Once you've learned to last, you'll recognize how close you are to having orgasms when you are on the edge of the pleasure plateau. From that point you can begin to fine-tune the experience through breath, awareness, and relaxation.

You are about to embark on a wonderfully fulfilling journey that is remarkably easy for most men. However, there are some men who need to see a specialist—whether it is a psychologist or urologist—for their problems related to premature ejaculation.

Start Your Training

To train yourself to last longer, you can practice by yourself or with your partner. The first step to training yourself is to engage your willpower. You will probably be tempted to just let go, as you always have, in order to achieve brief orgasmic pleasure. But rest assured that if you are willing to trust and back away from that point of no return a few times, whole new worlds will open to you and your lover. The training will also involve the following:

- Devoting some quality time to these fun training sessions.
- Learning to relax in the excitement of orgasmic bliss.
- Changing your habit of chest breathing to belly breathing.
- Learning simple communication practices with your partner.
- Loving your body and all the wonderful things it's capable of.

If you do this on your own, self-pleasure yourself until you reach an eight or nine (on the scale of one to ten) of your arousal. Stop, relax, and breathe deeply into your belly for a few minutes; then start again. Don't tense your body—relax it. This will require some self-restraint at first. Bring your focus and willpower to bear.

Tension in the body is typically what causes men to ejaculate. By voluntarily relaxing in the high state of arousal and combining that with slow, deep belly breathing, you will create a container for more powerful, long-lasting pleasure.

FACT

It's reported that up to 75 percent of all men ejaculate within two to five minutes of beginning intercourse. A survey of 1,370 men conducted by Tantra.com revealed that less than 35 percent felt they had any control over when they ejaculate.

If you have a partner, it is ideal to practice this together. The techniques are fun and will likely add a new dimension to lovemaking for many couples. It may be a rare experience for a woman to be handed the control button to her man. It may also require both of you to learn a lot of new hand job techniques for pleasuring. (You can refer to Chapter 15 for some of those strokes.)

Incorporate What You've Learned

You will very soon understand that as you master the ability to stop before going over the top, you will actually experience orgasmic-like pleasure without ejaculation. After a few weeks of practicing, you're going to want to try it out during intercourse with your partner.

Don't expect to be able to take your new-found control straight to coitus without a few hitches. You will have to start the process over, but it should be much easier this time. You'll have to stop at that eight or nine arousal point and rest. This time, though, your body and mind will be working together and they'll know what to do.

Know What Pleasures You

Changing positions, learning correct breathing, and controlling ejaculation will certainly help you enhance your orgasms as well as your lover's. But one often-overlooked and yet obvious point that needs to be made is that in order to fully enjoy yourself, you need to know what pleasures you. Take as many opportunities as possible to learn about your hot spots. What gets you juicy or aroused? Do words turn you on? How about teasing or seduction? Erotic dances from your lover? Small gifts? Tenderness?

Explore your body and how it prefers to be touched. Do you prefer soft caresses or to be squeezed and hugged? Do you prefer to be touched all over, or do you have specific areas that most desire touch? Do you like a single stimulation point, or can you handle two, three, or more? Do you like your nipples squeezed or your whole breast fondled with just a hint of nipple? Do you like your scrotum to be pulled firmly or cupped gently?

A person's preferences usually change from moment to moment. We'll like one thing this time and something else the next. But most of us find that we also have our favorite spots and secret desires when it comes to touch. The problem is, we keep them secret. Let your lover know what you like; but first, discover it for yourself. You won't be able to tell what you don't know.

Our genitals are most sensitive to touch, but there are other erogenous areas you may want to explore. Try combining one or two of these additional areas with genital stimulation. Vary the touch you give by using your fingertips, tickling, blowing, lightly scratching, or just holding the area. Learning to receive multiple types of touch will create more possibilities for orgasmic pleasure.

CHAPTER 12

Hot Spots and Sexual Taboos

The topic of taboos can be a tricky one to discuss, partly because the term can be a little hard to define. What one person (or couple) considers a taboo, others may consider nothing out of the ordinary. Cultural influences play a big role. In very conservative cultures, all but the most basic sexual activities may be considered taboo. Even the word taboo can have different connotations, depending on the person: for some, it's dirty and off-limits, for other it's naughty and exciting. Some taboo topics will be covered in this chapter. If you and your partner are both willing, try out a few, if you haven't already.

The G-Spot (or Goddess Spot)

It is widely believed that women have at least two vaginal areas that will respond to sexual arousal. One is located toward the back of the vaginal canal and closer to the cervix (the opening to the uterus). The other is the G-spot, an area located on the upper anterior wall of the vagina, about 1 to 1½ inches in, past the opening of the vagina and just behind the pubic bone. The G-spot lies between the two roots of the clitoris, which are buried under the skin and beneath the pubic bone. It consists of spongy material that is analogous to the prostate gland in men.

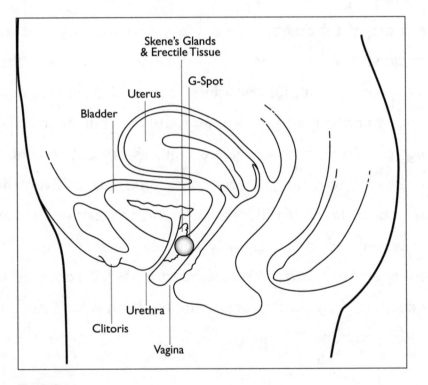

The G-Spot.

Exploring the Goddess Spot

Let's learn how to access your G-spot and what to expect when you do. By awakening the G-spot, you will have access to a whole new realm of orgasmic potential. Some women will find this exploration easy; for others, it will be a little more challenging. All sorts of emotional reactions—

including uncontrollable laughter—can occur when the spot is stimulated. Be prepared for anything!

QUESTION

Where did the term G-spot come from?
It's named after Ernst Grafenberg, the scientist who identified this sensitive area. In recent years, the G-spot has also been lovingly called the Goddess spot. Almost every woman has this spot or area, and most will be able to find it with a little training.

The benefits of awakening the G-spot will really show up during sexual intercourse. With a little practice you'll begin to recognize exactly where your G-spot is while in coitus, and that will enable you to subtly position yourself for just the right contact. Your G-spot awareness will be heightened, and you'll begin to notice it when you do your Kegel exercises and when you're making love. That will help you to empower your own orgasmic potential.

Exploration of a Partner's G-Spot

This section is written with the assumption that you and your partner will be doing this exploration together. The instructions are directed toward the man, unless otherwise indicated.

When you are preparing for this intimate exploration, you should both be relaxed. Take a bath or shower to help you get into a calm mood. Music, soft lighting, and a massage, if possible, can really help. Spend some time on a little foreplay. Get turned on. The woman may even want to have a clitoral orgasm. This will increase blood flow to the vulva and vagina and, as a consequence, to the G-spot.

Partners, here is where your role begins. Once you're both ready, use your middle finger to explore the G-spot, which is located less than two inches into the vagina just behind the pubic bone, on the top part of the woman's body. It helps if your finger is lubricated.

It's important to move slowly. As your finger enters the vagina, you'll feel the softness and then an area marked by its ridges. If you move your finger around, you'll notice that there really isn't any other area quite like the ridge area. Come back to that spot and proceed a tiny bit farther, just behind it to an indented space that is directly behind the pubic bone.

FACT

If you have been doing your Kegel exercises, your vaginal walls will have become tighter and the internal muscles will be stronger. This – and the increased sensitivity of that area will probably help you get in touch with your G-spot more easily. You've been stimulating it during the practice!

Apply very firm pressure. Your finger should be in a "hooked" or "come hither" position. Ask your partner what she is feeling. She may already be giving you some indications of sensations. Try slowly moving your finger in the "come hither" motion. Now try slowly sweeping your finger in a windshield washer motion. Is that different? Better? What does your partner like best? You may be amazed how much pressure this area can take. Don't be afraid to try applying more of it.

It is very important at these beginning stages to ask how your lover is doing. Encourage her to be clear with you about what she likes and doesn't like. If this is new territory for her, she is going to appreciate the questions and feel more confident about being able to guide you. She is discovering new things about her body, and if you can both stay open, connected, and in communication, you will both gain not just information, but a whole lot of pleasure.

Most men feel very empowered and successful as lovers when they help their partner discover her G-spot. While you shouldn't let this go to your head, do acknowledge yourself for being willing to help your lover know more about her body and expanding her pleasure potential.

What the Woman Can Expect

Many reactions can come up at this point during the joint G-spot exploration process. The woman may feel the urge to pee, she may feel a slight burning, she may feel pleasure, or she may feel a combination of any of these sensations. She may feel apprehensive, frightened, or even elated. She may laugh, cry, or cringe in perceived pain. Remember, this is a sensitive area!

Solo Exploration

If you are exploring this area by yourself, much of the same information applies. You should find a position that enables you to comfortably put your middle finger into your vagina and have enough latitude to move around some. Good positions for this are on your knees and sitting down a bit on your calves and on all fours with one hand free to explore. These positions bring your uterus down a bit and provide a better angle for your hand to have proper access.

Advanced Practice

The more you practice the finger methods, the more in touch you are going to be with your vagina and your G-spot. You are in the process of awakening a sleeping beauty! As this happens, see if you notice any changes in your awareness of your G-spot during intercourse. If you're doing your Kegel exercises daily, you should notice even more sensations.

In order to feel your G-spot better during intercourse, have your partner thrust slowly and shallowly at least half of the time. This will cause the head of the penis to rub the G-spot more frequently and produce more friction. Try various thrusting patterns like the following: nine shallow, one deep; eight shallow, two deep; seven shallow, three deep; and so forth.

Certain positions greatly benefit the stimulation of the G-spot. The "woman on top" and "rear-entry" positions are great for G-spot gratification.

And, finally, you are encouraged to make sounds. Practice making sounds that resonate from deep within your belly. You can do this while you are by yourself and then introduce it into your lovemaking later. Open your mouth and make low-register moans that don't come from your throat but from your abdomen. These kinds of sounds can bring on multiple G-spot orgasms.

Oral Sex

Although times are changing, some men and women have misgivings about both giving and receiving oral sex. Not all couples are comfortable with it and may need some encouragement in this area of lovemaking. Other couples already enjoy oral sex, but they may be able to use new information to improve their knowledge.

Some believe that oral sex was not common until the 1960s and 1970s, when it became wildly popular with the advent of women's magazines seeking yet another cutting-edge story for the cultural avant-garde. Today it has generally lost its taboo status; its appeal is enormous and lends great creativity and erotic pleasure to any relationship.

Oral sex is often considered an essential part of foreplay, but it can also be a very pleasurable stand-alone activity. Many women find that oral sex is the only way they can have an orgasm. While this book aims to help you expand your orgasmic potential, the fact that for many women it's the only way to go (or come!) points to the value of oral sex.

When preparing for this type of intimate contact, cleanliness is important. Bathe together, and pay close attention to the little details. Men, if you aren't circumcised, pay special attention to the area under your foreskin. Women, wash with a gentle but effective soap. You'll both be more comfortable and relaxed knowing that you are clean and prepared.

Stimulating the Clitoris

Clitorises come in many sizes, but they are small in relationship to the rest of a woman's sexual organs. The clitoris is covered by a piece of skin or hood that protects it from being rubbed or irritated during most of the day. The head and the hood are the exterior parts of the clitoris, but there is much more buried under the skin, past the head.

As the woman gets more turned on, the clitoris begins to fill with blood and become engorged. This causes the clitoris to become erect. As this happens, the head of the clitoris "hides" up under the hood more. It's often useful for the woman to help out by holding the hood that covers the clitoris back, out of the way for her lover.

When it comes to oral sex on a woman, you need to be subtle but focused. Pick one area you think is most sensitive and then stick with one speed and one kind of movement for a while. The giver has to develop the stamina required for repetitive movements like these.

It's useful to know that most women have a particular area of their clitoris that is most sensitive. This doesn't mean that it all doesn't feel good, but one area is usually the most sensitive. Most women find that stimulation of the top of their clitoris is the most pleasurable.

You also need to pay some attention to the labia, or lips of the vulva, which are sensitive to touch and licking. Start with the labia and slowly move in to focus on the clitoris after the outer areas have had some attention. You can gently suck, lick, blow softly, and nibble on any of these parts.

ALERT

Warning: never blow air inside a woman's vagina. In rare cases, this can cause an air bubble to enter the body—and if it goes into your bloodstream, that can be dangerous or even deadly. Aside from that issue, the sensation of air entering the vagina is usually just plain uncomfortable.

Try different modalities of touch with your lips, tongue, tip of the tongue, and even teeth if you are very careful. Be very tender in your touch.

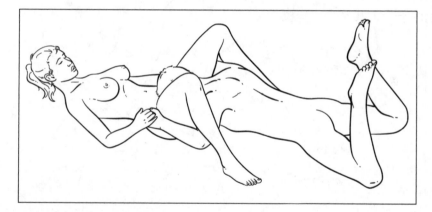

Woman receiving oral sex.

Women, when you're receiving oral sex, remember to relax as you get more and more turned on. Breathe deeply and stay aware of your body and what is happening. As you become more turned on, you may notice that you begin to curl up a little. Your stomach, hips, and buttocks tighten up. When you find yourself tensing up, relax again. If you allow your body to curl, the clitoris only becomes more hidden and harder for your partner to stimulate. Open your body up and out, and breathe. This will expand your orgasmic potential.

Many women instinctively keep their legs close together while receiving oral sex, but by opening her legs as wide as possible, she gives her partner access to more areas of her body (and also makes it easier for herself or her partner to stimulate manually at the same time).

Also, by putting her legs up in the air (pulling them back with her hands, if needed) or bringing her knees to her chest, the woman allows the man to have deeper penetration and easier access to her clitoris.

Some couples like to engage in cunnilingus with the man lying on his back and the woman straddling his face.

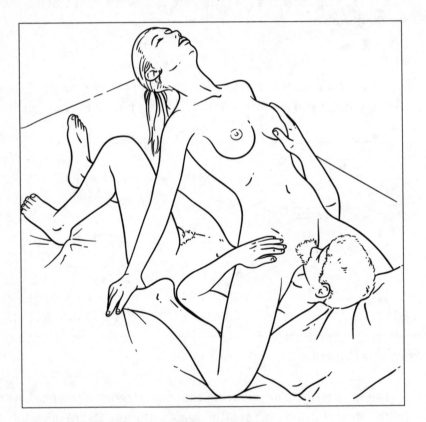

Cunnilingus with woman straddling man's face.

Stimulating the Penis

Receiving oral sex is sometimes the most fantasized part of the sexual experience for men. Many men have seen pornography that portrays women giving oral sex with wild abandon. They consider it erotic and intimate for their lover to give them fellatio, to ejaculate into their lover's mouth, and to have the lover swallow their ejaculate.

ESSENTIAL

Remember, women, it's not about taking him over the top too quickly. Train him by getting to know his arousal patterns and then backing off when he's getting close to ejaculating. This training can come in handy when you are having intercourse and you both want him to last longer.

It's wonderful to start with a soft penis. This allows the exquisite feeling of having the man respond in your mouth to the touch you are giving. As you begin, touch your partner tenderly with your hands and gently blow on his pubic area. Cup his scrotum in your hands and carefully fondle the hair and skin around his genitals. Begin to kiss and lick his shaft. Start out with more of a teasing touch. As he warms up, move to a firmer touch.

Once the penis begins to grow, move to the head. As you prepare to take it in, make sure your mouth is very wet. Play with him in a teasing manner as you go back and forth from his shaft to the head and back again, kissing, sucking, and even very lightly biting as you move up the shaft to the head of his penis.

Once he is very aroused, begin to take more control and be more aggressive. Stay on the head longer and with more regular strokes of your mouth. If you feel comfortable, use the technique called *deep throating* to take his penis deeper into your mouth. Be careful and go slowly—he'll like it better that way. Pay particular attention to the head and the edge where it meets the shaft. This area is very sensitive in most men, and he'll love the attention you give to it.

Many men like increased stimulation as they get further aroused. They tend to like a series of repetitive actions and strokes. Vary the intensity so that you have a sense of where your partner is in his arousal state. By beginning to create a kind of dance with softer, more sensual strokes to hotter, firmer suction, you'll be able to help train your man to last longer.

There are several types of positions that can be used in giving fellatio:

- Some women are fine performing oral sex while kneeling on the floor with the man standing in front of them.

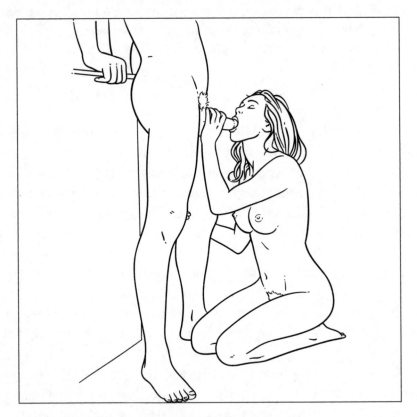

Woman performing oral sex while kneeling on floor.

- Other women find kneeling on the floor uncomfortable and prefer to kneel on a bed or lie on their stomachs, while the man lies near them or stands against the bed in front.

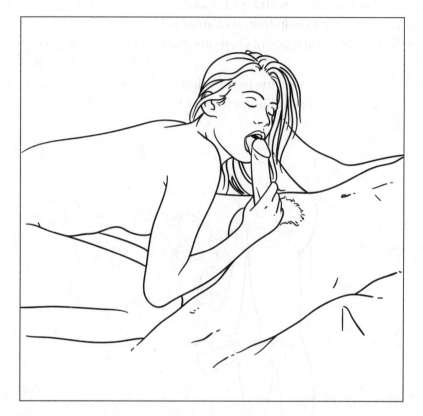

Woman performing oral while kneeling on bed.

- Still another variation involves the woman lying on her back, with the man hovering above her, with his legs apart. This provides the woman with access to the man's scrotum and other areas, while also giving the man the opportunity to reach down and caress the woman's breasts. Should the woman decide to use one hand to masturbate, the man would also have a great view of the action.

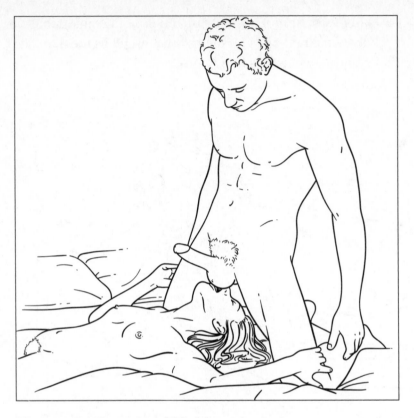

Woman performing oral sex while lying on her back.

Turn Up the Heat

To take oral sex up another level, you can add in stimulation with your hands or breasts. Encourage your partner to receive more pleasure by stimulating other parts of his body as you're performing oral sex. Or you can ask your lover to touch you as you're doing it.

Caressing, teasing, rubbing, biting, blowing, pulling, cupping, even scratching lightly—all these things and more will add to the overall pleasure during oral sex. Try gently pulling the pubic hair around your lover's genitals. Comb your fingers through the pubic hair and use your hands to pleasure the breasts and nipples; rub your breasts across his legs as you take his penis into your mouth.

Here are a few other fun suggestions:

- Try humming while engaged in oral sex. Gently vibrate the lips to add the sensation to both the vulva and the penis.
- See how it feels to give and receive oral sex while standing or kneeling. Men will often get harder when they are standing or kneeling.
- Relax into an overstuffed chair while engaging in oral sex. This works for either partner and keeps the neck of the giver from cramping.
- Many couples think the position 69 (with both partners giving each other oral sex at the same time) is the ultimate. It is sometimes difficult for women to receive a gentler touch because the man will often want a faster, firmer stroke. But both partners tend to melt into a similar speed and touch when in 69.

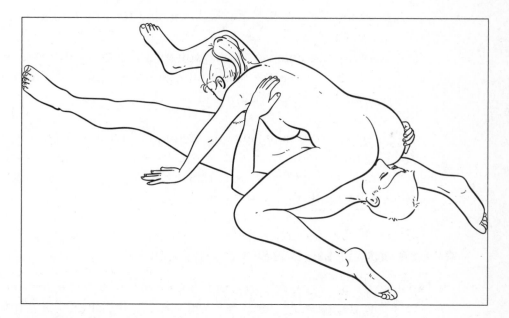

The "69" position.

- Use ice cubes, warm liquids or liquors, or edible body butters for an added turn on. These may also be a great way to introduce a reluctant partner into trying oral sex.

ESSENTIAL

Never coerce reluctant partners into doing anything that they feel isn't right for them. Do encourage them to talk about their feelings and attitudes about the subject, and do express your own feelings, but don't try to convince them to change.

Communication Is Key

As you explore oral sex, ask for your partner's feedback. If you're the giver, pay attention to what your partner is saying. If you're the receiver, don't just assume your partner knows your body or your mind. If you need help expressing yourself, use this simple communication technique:

1. Say something you like that is happening right then: "I love the speed you are using."
2. Ask for a single change: "Would you try moving slightly to the left?"
3. Give some kind of a response: "Ah, thank you, that's great" or "Oh, that's not as good as I thought it would be."

This simple communication technique includes an acknowledgement, a single change, and a response. This can be used over and over to get the kind of touch that you love. It's training for your partner and for you to know exactly what it is that turns you on!

Anal Stimulation and Anal Sex

Anal sexual activity is a taboo subject for many people. Yet, just as oral sex was a few decades ago, anal sex and other forms of anal play have come into more favor in recent years.

One partner is often more eager and/or curious to try anal sex than the other. If your partner is willing to try, great. But if not, you may suggest experimenting with other types of anal stimulation. The truth is that the anus and the area around it are full of nerve endings. There are a variety of things you and your partner can do to stimulate these areas besides anal intercourse.

Pleasurable attention to the anus can lead both of you to much stronger orgasms and sexual ecstasy.

Women will like stimulation of the anus toward the area of the G-spot. The membrane between the anus and the vagina is very thin. Combining anal and G-spot stimulation adds to the sensual feeling for women.

Because the G-spot is analogous to the prostate gland, men will like this upper area also. Feel for the prostate gland. Hold pressure here when stimulating the man.

Finger Play

There's no reason to rush. Begin by talking about any beliefs or hesitations you might have with your partner. If you both agree to try some anal play, keep it simple, and communicate with each other while you are experimenting. Don't expect too much at first, and have the receiving partner be in complete control of the situation.

It's best if your first few experiences are limited to finger play. Before you begin, take a bath to get clean and relaxed. Open your partner up by massaging and being playful.

Introduce anal play by lubricating a finger and playing with the area immediately around the anus before moving toward the opening. Slowly and gently add a little stimulation without entering. Ask your partner if he is ready for you to enter. If you get permission, slowly and sensually insert one finger.

ESSENTIAL

Latex gloves can be essential to have on hand for things like anal play. Keep gloves, finger cots, and condoms around for such occasions. They can add a sense of fantasy, play, and safety to your sexual exploring.

It's helpful if you are both turned on before anal play starts. Men, try giving your partner oral sex first and ask her if you can enter her with one finger as she is close to orgasm and after you have stimulated the outer area of her anus. The same applies for men. He should be turned on first—he will be much more accepting of penetration.

Anal Sex

Try experimenting with some anal toys before you have anal intercourse. Women may love having a small, soft anal plug inside them while having vaginal intercourse. Men, you'll love the tighter fit, too.

If you're ready for anal sex, be sure to use lots of water-based lubricant, because the anal cavity doesn't self-lubricate. And unless you are monogamous and both of you are HIV negative, use a condom during anal intercourse.

Before you begin, massage and warm your partner's anal area. Make sure she's relaxed and ready. The woman's anus will actually relax and open if you go slowly and let her set the pace. Place the head of your penis at the entrance and allow her to move toward you.

Good positions to start are with the woman on her back with her legs up and the man on his knees.

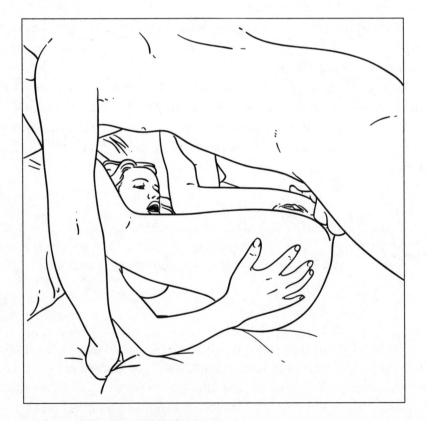

Anal sex, with woman on her back.

Rear entry works well, but don't try this the first time you have anal sex, because the woman is less in control in rear-entry positions.

A good anal sex position, especially for couples who are first experimenting with this activity, is for the man and woman to lie on their sides, with the man behind the woman. This generally makes frantic thrusting difficult, which may put the woman more at ease.

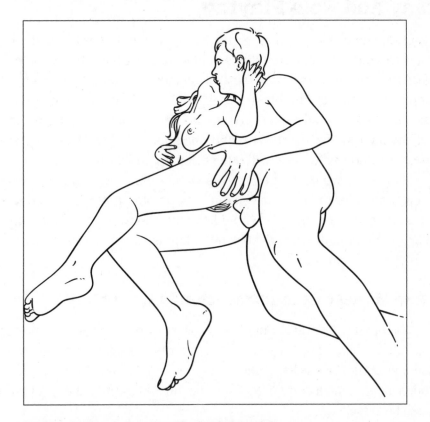

Anal sex, with man lying on side behind woman.

ALERT

Never put a finger, hand, penis, dildo, vibrator, or anything else into the vagina if it has just been in the rectum or anus. This can cause the woman to get a vaginal infection. Always wash anything that has been in the anus very thoroughly before inserting it into the vagina.

Remember, don't ever coerce or force your partner into anything he doesn't want to do. Learning to relax into anal stimulation is healthy. The anus and buttocks area holds a lot of tension and stress. It is to our advantage to learn to relax that region, both physically and emotionally.

Fantasy and Role Playing

Games, role-playing, and recreating some of your fantasies together can add new excitement and possibilities to maturing relationships. People make up fantasies because even the best of relationships needs new stimulus and input. The subject of fantasy is a whole book in itself. Everyone has fantasies. Even if you think you don't, you do have desires, and desires are a form of fantasy, too. We are creative and imaginative beings. When we feel cared for, safe, and trusting, we will often open up about our fantasy life.

Fantasies are best when they're shared. Sharing fantasies can open up new realms for many couples. You may be pleasantly surprised to find out that your partner secretly wanted to try something that you wanted, too. Or, you might find yourself starting to fantasize about something once your partner mentions it.

Open and Honest Communication Is Important

Be open to talking about your fantasies, starting out slowly and sensitively and then building up over time to some of the edgier ones. Keep a healthy perspective on what is doable and what is not. And don't assume that just because you find a certain fantasy to be fun and exciting that your partner will feel the same way.

Don't Be Too Judgmental

Keep an open mind when it comes to listening to your partner's fantasies. He may have needed to muster up a lot of courage in order to reveal this fantasy to you, and if you react negatively he may be reluctant to share other private things with you in the future. You can decline to engage in a particular fantasy in a gentle and nonjudgmental way. Simply say it's not your cup of tea. If possible, come up with a variation that's more enjoyable to you.

Even if you are a bit shocked by your partner's fantasy, try not to react with horror. If you really don't know how to react or if you need time to digest the information, a good stalling technique is to provide a distraction by mentioning a fantasy of your own. Who knows—once you've had time to really contemplate your partner's fantasy, you might find yourself warming up to the idea.

Role Playing

Role playing is basically like taking fantasies to the next level. You and your partner are acting out your fantasies together in a fun and exciting way. Even the best relationships can fall into a rut after a while, so role playing can be a great way to spice things up, especially for couples who are in a long-term relationship and are eager to try something new and different.

ESSENTIAL

With role playing, just as with fantasies, it is very important that you be receptive and open-minded toward your partner's ideas. If you really aren't into the specific scenario your partner mentions, try to suggest a compromise or alternative that you'd both enjoy.

The role playing scenarios you can choose are limited only by your imagination and your tastes. With enough creativity (and some helpful outfits and/or props) you can act out virtually any roles you can imagine. You can start with the old stand-by scenarios—student/teacher, boss/secretary, etc.—and then move on to more outrageous ones. Consider it a challenge to see just how original you can be!

Swings, Velvet Handcuffs, and More

There are whole categories of extras that many couples enjoy to spice up their relationships. Make sure both of you are in agreement before acting on your fantasies and desires. The most important thing is to have fun.

There are several varieties of love swings on the market. They are versatile, fun, and add variations to lovemaking positions. Love swings aid in G-spot stimulation and can be helpful for men interested in learning to last longer. They can be hung in a variety of places in the house and the yard as the imagination dictates.

If you are interested in playing with light bondage or S-M, there are books and DVDs specifically devoted to the subject. Do some research together and discuss it before you agree to try this type of activity. Communication and trust are of the utmost importance, and you need to know how to approach the activities with care and knowledge. Couples may find new realms open to them through experiences such as these.

X-Rated Films

If you don't have much experience with X-rated films, you may envision them to be gross, disturbing, or even a bit scary. Before jumping to conclusions, though, you should really check out some adult movies for yourself. Give them a fair chance. It's very important to try a few different types of films, preferably from a variety of companies and/or producers. Just as with mainstream films, adult films come in many different styles and genres. There are the more romantic style that are often described with terms like "erotic" and "sensual." On the other end of the spectrum are the hardcore and graphic varieties that are geared toward the more adventurous viewers. Then there are soft-core porn films that tend to be a little tamer and often only show partial nudity.

ESSENTIAL

A popular trend in adult films is the increase in erotic movies that are made by women, for women. These tend to have a little more dialogue and more storyline that the typical adult film, and they often spend more time on scenes featuring foreplay.

Many people are intimated by adult films because they fear that they (or their bodies) won't "measure up" when compared to the actors on screen. Relax! Most likely, your partner is turned on by what the actors are doing, not necessarily what they look like.

If you find it distracting to compare yourself to the perfect-looking film stars, a good solution can be to try watching amateur adult films. These are made by real people, with real (usually unenhanced) bodies.

Pornography

In addition to adult movies, there is also the old-school type of pornography: magazines and pictures. These can be a way to become comfortable with adult images and ease your way into the material before you check out some X-rated films. Just as with films, these types of materials run the gamut from tame to wild. Again, it's a good idea to check out a few different types to find the styles that you and your partner like best.

Porn Preferences

While plenty of people enjoy looking at adult magazines and erotic pictures, others find that these inactive images just don't do anything for them. Many people find it much more exciting to watch the scenes on screen so they can see and hear every aspect of the action. Fortunately, there are so many options available that you can take your pick.

When Is Porn a Problem?

For many couples, adult materials can be a great way to enhance their sex lives and bring some added excitement to the bedroom. But occasionally these materials can cause problems for one or both members of a couple. Some red flags:

- If you and/or your partner find it impossible to become aroused without the use of adult materials
- If one of you begins hiding your adult materials and covertly using them behind the other's back
- If one of you starts spending so much time viewing porn that your real-life sex life as a couple suffers

If any of these or other porn-related problems becomes an issue for you, it's probably time for you and your partner to have a serious discussion about porn's role in your relationship. In extreme cases, it might be necessary to enlist the help of a therapist or counselor.

CHAPTER 13

Aphrodisiacs and Sexual Aids

While porn can be a great way to add sizzle to your sex life, there are plenty of other helpful items that can make things fresh and exciting in the bedroom. You can enhance your sexual experience with special foods, toys, adult gadgets, props, and more. Really, just about anything can be used as a bedroom aid if you have enough imagination (and, in some cases, adventurousness). In fact, it can be fun to take something innocent or unusual and try to find an erotic use for it. Experiment and be creative!

The Power of Aphrodisiacs

An aphrodisiac is a substance (generally, a food or drink) that you use to enhance pleasure or susceptibility to pleasure. The list of possible aphrodisiacs is probably endless, since everyone's tastes are different. Plus, a substance can have aphrodisiac effects if it reminds someone of an enjoyable experience. Many people become aroused when exposed to certain foods, odors, or environments that their brain associates with sex.

Sensual foods have a definite place in the bedroom. They are especially welcome if they are juicy, soft, mysterious, and sweet. If the foods are evocative reminders of sexual organs, there's even more reason to include them as part of your lovemaking ritual.

You can have lots of fun with food in the bedroom. Food can be used for stimulating the various senses. Try an evening of lovemaking that involves blindfolding your partner and offering her different sorts of fruits, chocolates, and desserts that are suggestive of softness or juiciness. This is more about sensing than it is about eating. Keep the bites very small and offer the food gently for smelling and brushing across the lips first, before letting your partner take the bite into her mouth.

Whipped cream and chocolate syrup are fun (though messy!) in the bedroom, but allowing these types of substances to dry and remain on the skin—or in/near bodily openings—can cause all sorts of problems. A good solution: enjoy a shower together after a food-enhanced sexual romp.

FACT

Some of the most well-publicized aphrodisiacs in ancient times were rhinoceros horn, elk antler, and powdered sea horse. There is little evidence that these substances actually work, however, and serious damage is being done to the environment today by people who want to obtain these aphrodisiacs.

Some substances that are commonly believed to have aphrodisiac qualities are oysters, chocolate, and wine. Certain spices and plants are also said to be aphrodisiacs.

While the stereotypical aphrodisiacs may indeed have an erotic effect on you, it can be fun to try to find new and unusual alternatives. Try lots of different foods, and you just may discover some exciting new arousal boosters.

Pheromones: The Chemicals of Love

Pheromones are chemicals found in body secretions that attract the opposite sex. They don't have a discernable smell, but humans have special detectors in their noses for pheromones. We respond physiologically to another person's pheromones, even if we cannot consciously smell them.

FACT

Pheromones are available for purchase; you can add them to your favorite perfume or dab them on separately. The jury is out on their effectiveness, since there haven't been many studies done with manufactured pheromones, but they aren't too expensive, so try some out for yourself.

The word *pheromone* is derived from a Greek word meaning "to transfer excitement." Body temperature, skin conductance, heart rate, and blood pressure are just some of the functions that can be affected by our reactions to our partner's pheromones. (Women taking oral contraceptives seem to be less responsive to pheromones.) Pheromones have also been isolated as the cause for synchronized menstruation cycles among women who live in close proximity over a period of time.

Male and female pheromones are excreted from glands in the hair follicles, the underarms, and the groin area. Some men and women are greatly attracted to the smell of their partners' underarms and hair. Try burying your nose in your partner's hair the next time you want to become aroused.

Scents and Perfumes

Scents and perfumes have been used since time immemorial, possibly to mimic pheromones. One of the most popular is musk, which has a smell very close to the male hormone testosterone. The Romans used civet and ambergris as the carriers for lavish perfumes that were erotic in nature.

Vanilla, lavender, and flower essences have been used for thousands of years to add allure to our bodily scents. Many of the tropical forests in Hawaii were cut down in the eighteenth and nineteenth centuries for the delicate, earthy scent of sandalwood. The finest European fans for aristocratic women were made from sandalwood. This wood never loses its scent, so it served as a perfume when a woman seductively fanned herself.

When choosing a perfume, pick something that isn't too overbearing. It should complement the subtle scent of your own skin, hair, and phero-mones. Try going without perfume sometimes, especially before a night of lovemaking. This way, it won't cover up your own natural erotic smells.

People have long used incense to set the scene for romance. Again, pick something that is appropriate and not overbearing. You might want to place it in an adjacent room like a bathroom so that the hint of it reaches you; you wouldn't want to be distracted by the full strength of the incense. You can also freshen a room by lighting incense and then putting it out quickly, to give just a hint of the scent.

By visiting an aromatherapy store, you can mix your own unique blend of oils and substances, thus creating a scent that is completely custom tai-lored to your own tastes. You may want to save this for special occasions, or perhaps to use as a secret signal (dab it on when you want your partner to know you're in the mood for love).

Just as with aphrodisiacs, scents can be a matter of personal tastes and preferences. One person may find a scent exciting, but it might be a turn-off for someone else. Don't worry if you get excited by an unusual scent (say, peanut butter or the smell of a new car). You're just unique!

Gels, Creams, and Lotions

Gels, creams, and lotions have become increasingly popular as sexual enhancers. This is partly because there are so many new and exciting variet-ies. You can choose from flavored and/or scented substances, varieties that warm up when exposed to body heat or friction, and even ones that claim to have extra arousal-stimulating ingredients. These substances also have a practical benefit: their lubricating properties make some sex acts more com-fortable or pleasurable.

Pay attention to the ingredients in your lotions of gels, especially if you are allergy prone and tend to have a negative reaction to certain chemicals, flavors, or scents. You must also remember that petroleum-based substances can be detrimental to condoms and other protective materials.

Massage oils and lotions can be great for a sensual massage, but they aren't designed to go inside the body (unless they are specifically labeled that way).

Check if the lubricant you are selecting has nonoxynol-9 in it. This additive is a spermicide, meaning it kills sperm. If you do not need the protection for pregnancy prevention, it is recommended you don't use these products. It can be irritating or cause an allergic reaction.

Heightening Creams

There are many new creams on the market that are designed with women in mind. Like Viagra does for men, these products are supposed to help with the physical aspects of sexual dysfunction that some women have in achieving orgasmic states.

FACT

In the first clinical trials that gave Viagra to women, fewer than 45 percent of the women had any positive response. A separate group determined that if the women were first screened for psychological problems and those subjects were removed, the remaining group of women who exhibited physical symptoms had a success rate of more than 90 percent.

The general function of these creams is to increase blood flow to the genitals. Blood flow causes the engorgement and arousal of the genital region. Many of these creams are based on the absorption of L-arginine into the blood supply in the immediate area of the genitals. L-arginine increases the nitric oxide available to the tissue, which in turn expands the blood vessels and allows more blood to flow to the region.

The creams that are currently on the market have varying degrees of success. This is a new area in the understanding of sexual response, and it is in its infancy. We can expect more of these products to be available in the coming years.

Lovemaking and Food

It's often been said that food is the way to a man's heart. Well, that can have a lot of different implications. Healthy eating is of course the optimum for all of us. But certain foods can have a positive effect on the libido.

Before we go on to examine what foods are compatible with the act of making love, a word of warning. Overeating before an evening of lovemaking can have a less-than-beneficial effect—both on the libido and on performance. Have you ever eaten a large meal and then had to go back to work and engage your brain for some critical thinking? The brain will often fail you in these times because the body has sent a lot of the blood supply to the stomach to aid in digestion. When we eat a meal, the blood flows away from the brain, away from the extremities, and away from the genitals.

ESSENTIAL

Make a short list of edible items you know increase your desire and libido. Share this list with your lover and ask her to do the same. Notice the things that are the same and the ones that are different.

Time for Food, Time for Love

If you are planning an evening of lovemaking that includes food, make eating a part of the ritual or ceremony of loving. That way, you can include eating in the sensual evening without stopping the action. Eating can be a fun addition. You can feed each other. Eat in courses so that eating takes a long time and is spread out between the courses of love.

Serving things like sushi, light pastas, small skewers of vegetables and fish, or a salad with many goodies in it. Then dessert could come later.

Maybe you present dessert on your inner thighs or you offer your partner the opportunity to become the platter. Find unique and fun ways to surprise yourself and your lover.

Suggestive Shapes

Try forming foods into shapes that are suggestive or downright sexual— you can use chocolates, little cakes, oysters, candies, breads, and main dishes. Your imagination can take you anywhere. Soak dried fruit in wine or liquors to enhance their flavor. Use fresh and dried fruit to dip into sauces that are sweetened and have a yogurt base. Dip fresh fruit into chocolate or butterscotch sauces. Raspberry sauce, whipped cream, and even ice cream can be used in erotic ways to enhance an evening of love.

Spice Up Your Life

Some spices, seasonings, and foods with certain amino acids are good for getting the heat to rise. Adding a variety of spices to your food concoctions can have a wonderful effect of heightening arousal. Pumpkin pie spices, licorice, cinnamon, peppermint, curries, coriander, cardamom, lavender, chili peppers, sesame seeds, saffron, nutmeg, and pepper—all these are believed to intensify sexual desire. They are generally also very good for your health and vitality.

Ginger, onions, and garlic are also considered aphrodisiacs by many cultures, as are asparagus, figs, grapes, almonds, oysters, mussels, caviar, basil, bananas, and mangos—the list goes on. Remember, anything can be erotic, and different people find different foods erotic. With this in mind, be sure to create foods that appeal to both you and your lover. It's fun creating and discovering new things together, and the time spent attending to the details will be well worth it.

Chocolate Temptation

One of the active ingredients in chocolate produces phenylethylamine, the chemical that the body manufactures when we fall in love. These chemical messengers speed up the flow of information that travels between our nerve endings. Phenylethylamine is similar in many ways to amphetamine, which dilates the blood vessels and creates energy and focus. It is not by chance that chocolate is so highly associated with love.

FACT

The Aztec emperor Montezuma was reported to have drunk up to fifty cups a day of chocolate with chili and spices in it. He had to keep up his stamina to satisfy his many wives! Some women crave chocolate as their hormonal balance shifts. Their subconscious thinks of it as a remedy to lift spirits and provide energy.

In Drunken Bliss

Used in moderation, alcohol can enhance the sensual or sexual experience. It can relax you and ease your inhibitions. In small amounts, it has been cited as an aid in helping men last longer so they don't ejaculate too fast. However, be aware that in larger amounts, it has the opposite effect.

Try using it in a ritual way by creating a ceremony when you drink it. Sip it during lovemaking. Share a kiss with a little liquor in your mouth and let it dribble down your cheeks.

Take some liquor into your mouth and then give your partner oral sex while you still have it in your mouth. Throw in the element of surprise. This can add new sensations to both your experiences. It can be licked and sucked off if any gets away from you!

Erotic Reading and Writing

Reading erotic materials to your partner can be exquisitely sensuous. As you read, you can place your own intention and inflection on the sentences you want to emphasize. You can even act out some of the parts and discuss or fantasize about what you are reading together.

Pillow books are books that have pictures, writing, and sometimes instructions—like position books. These provide a great resource for erotic adventure. There are several ancient erotic pillow books that not only brought pleasure, but also helped educate people over many generations. These books are available today in modern forms and are informative, evocative, and titillating.

If you are inclined to write a love letter but feel intimidated, ask for help at the bookstore. Purchase a book of poetry by Rumi or another love poet and generously sprinkle some of their words in your letter. It'll turn your partner on in more than one way!

Writing poetry has long been a symbol of both romantic and erotic love. Even writers of little skill can successfully write poetry to their lover that will be received as though it came from a master. The gift of writing is a gift of time, care, and love. Read and write poetry together. Try writing one poem together and see what you come up with.

Even if poetry isn't something that turns you on, consider stretching yourself a little if it is something you think your lover would like. In addition, write little love notes that point to the anticipation of a particular erotic event that you have planned. Leading up to a date with notes and love letters is an outrageous way to create titillating tension. By the time you get together, you'll be all over each other!

Words of Love and Lust

For both men and women, words can be powerful erotic stimulators. In general, men will prefer lusty, teasing, more explicitly sexual language. Women tend to respond to more indirect language—hints, words of love and desire, and compliments. Regardless of what you like, the idea is to start the erotic play before you get to the bedroom. The longer we are juiced up, the stronger our reactions will be when we get there.

Don't hesitate to use words liberally when making love and make sounds to let your partner know how you are feeling. Here's an activity to try. It has several different variations. You may want to create new additional versions that are appropriate for times other than when you are making love. Sit facing each other when you do these, and take turns.

- Give each other the gift of one minute of compliments. Just say loving, complimentary words and phrases as they come to your mind. Don't think too much—just let them flow.

- Each of you takes one minute to say as many erotic, hot, sexy words as you can come up with. Don't censor your words—just let them out.
- In one minute, say words of compassion, care, and sympathy as they come to your mind. Use this one when one or both of you are experiencing hurt or vulnerability.
- Use words of gratitude and thanks for one minute each. This practice helps us remember to speak about how precious our lives are. Use this one generously!
- Make up your own version with themes that fit your life.

Between the Sheets

There are a lot of toys and other sexual aids that can be very useful during sex. If you haven't tried some of these products, talk with your partner about purchasing the ones that intrigue the two of you. If you are single, you're sure to find something on this list that titillates you.

Vibrators

Vibrators are excellent for women who need help learning to orgasm. If a woman has been frustrated with her capacity to have orgasms, using a vibrator can open the door to that experience. Start with a small one designed for clitoral stimulation.

Some women like vibrators, while others prefer dildos, which are used inside the vagina. You can also purchase a vibrating dildo. You may need to explore a few to discover what works for you. Each type has a specific purpose.

If you have a partner, talk to him about going to an adult store to look over the selection. Be sensitive to your lover's feelings about this. He may have feelings of inadequacy at not being the lover you want him to be. Reassure him that you only want to add to the repertoire of your adventures in bed.

Vibrators do have a downside—they can be addictive and desensitizing. Your lover may find that you are having a harder time reaching orgasm when he is giving you oral stimulation, if you have been using the vibrator a lot. Pay attention and modify its use if this seems to be a problem. Vibrators can be great to use during intercourse to stimulate the woman's clitoris. Either partner can hold it and add to the pleasure.

Men may have an interest in some of the sensations a vibrator has to offer. Try the small clitoral vibrators on the perineum during intercourse or while giving him oral sex. This is healthy stimulation and exercise for the prostate gland, too. It may stimulate more sexual excitement or may defocus the intensity, which helps to delay orgasm and ejaculation in men.

Dildos

Dildos come in all shapes, sizes, materials, and forms. There are combinations for stimulating the clitoris and for insertion into the vagina; there are ones just for the vagina; there are anal plugs for anal stimulation; and there are combinations for vagina and anus. Some will be battery-operated vibrators, and some will be without vibration. And in each of these categories there are literally hundreds of varieties.

There are so many options to choose from. Go to a well-equipped website or adult store when you make your first purchases. Websites are great to browse and order from because they offer privacy and ease.

Condoms and Gloves

Condoms, gloves, and other latex products can be fun to use, even for committed, monogamous couples who are free of sexually transmitted diseases. Even if you are in a long-term relationship and can safely have unprotected sex, try using a condom once in a while. They may fit into sexual fantasies for you or just be fun to try. The same goes for gloves. The use of latex gloves adds a fantasy dimension to lovemaking and they work very well for anal stimulation for both men and women. They can take the edge off trying these things if you are new to this kind of sexual exploring.

Sexual Response Remedies

There are numerous products and substances that are promoted specifically to help boost a less-than-optimal sexual response. Here are some natural varieties:

- **Ginkgo biloba and ginseng.** Both are recommended for improving blood flow to the brain and extremities. Ginkgo greatly increases the concentrations of dopamine and other neurotransmitters, the forerunners of increased pleasure, happiness, and alertness. Ginseng increases the production of sex hormones like testosterone and progesterone and helps keep up your stamina. It helps moderate stress, stimulates the immune system, and can decrease menopausal symptoms.

- **Lycium fruit.** This Chinese berry has been used as a natural treatment for male impotence, as well as health conditions such as anemia and lung problems.

- **Saw palmetto.** This herb is effective in stopping swollen prostate growth. While some claim that it can actually shrink a swollen prostate gland, most experts say that it is effective only in stopping additional swelling from occurring. This can help increase the flow of semen from the testicles, help with urinary problems in older men, and relieve the tension to the urinary tract caused by the enlarged gland. This tension often leads to an uncomfortable feeling during sex. Since men over age fifty are so susceptible to prostate enlargement, it is a good idea to take saw palmetto regularly as a preventative measure.

- **Black cohosh.** This herb is known for its balancing effect on female hormones. Both estrogen and progesterone levels are influenced by its properties. It is a great treatment for premenstrual symptoms and menopausal problems related to lubrication and sexual receptiveness.

In addition to these natural substances, there are a few more supplements worth mentioning. Wild yam, L-arginine (taken orally), kava kava, Damiana, Pygeum, and stinging nettle are a few. You can find more information on these items and others in books, on the Internet, and from reliable health food stores. Not only are they healthful additives to your diet, they have the added distinction of whetting your sexual appetite.

Viagra and Other Sexual Enhancement Drugs

Lagging libidos have become big business for large pharmaceutical companies. It seems there's been a whole new crop of these drugs hitting the marketplace just in the past few years. In a way, this is good news, because it means more men are taking steps to address their sexual issues, whereas in the past they may have just suffered in silence and learned to live with it. Still, some experts believe that the vast majority of erectile dysfunction goes undiagnosed.

Viagra

Probably the most well-known of the sexual enhancement drugs is Viagra. It is the most widely prescribed drug for male erectile dysfunction. The pills are easily recognizable, thanks to their blue color and diamond shape.

Just a reminder: Prescription drugs used to treat sexual problems can have negative interactions with other medications. Before you take Viagra or a similar drug, make sure to tell your doctor about any other medications (both prescription and over-the-counter) you take, to avoid any serious problems.

ALERT

While there are several drugs to help treat impotence and a slow libido, there are also a number of drugs that can sometimes cause these conditions. Common culprits include diuretics, anti-depressants, and blood pressure medications. Alcohol and street drugs can also have negative effects on your sex drive.

Natural Viagra?

Recently, there's been a trend in which stores—especially online shops—will tout certain herbs or other substances as natural Viagra. Take these claims with a big grain of salt and a lot of caution. At best, the claims of these substances' sexual powers are probably greatly exaggerated. Worse, these substances can be potentially dangerous.

Unlike prescription medications, herbs and supplements don't have to be evaluated by the Food and Drug Administration or any other regulatory agency.

Female Viagra?

With all this attention focused on Viagra and similar drugs for men, many women have been demanding a similar magic pill that can work wonders for them in the bedroom. Alas, that seems to be a way off in the future. Several drug companies have claimed to be in the process of developing a drug that will help improve women's experiences, but so far no such wonder drug has hit the market.

CHAPTER 14

Tantra, *Kama Sutra*, and More

Sex has been around as long as people have, so it's not surprising that our ancestors have some time-tested wisdom to share on the subject. Even in this modern age, many people still look to the ancient sex guides to discover new sensual techniques. Books like the *Kama Sutra*, written centuries ago, continue to serve as part inspiration and part education for many current-day lovers. Check them out—you might be surprised!

Anicent and Modern Tantra

Tantra originates from India, where it has been practiced for thousands of years. Tantric practices were at their height between A.D. 500 and 1300. The spiritual, sexual, and personal transformative components of tantra include whole-body health and Ayurvedic medicine. Today, it remains a living system that is designed to promote rapid growth toward enlightenment in the individual.

In India, not everyone has the honor of studying tantra. In order to practice it, you must have a guru who deems you worthy of this art. In tantra, elaborate rituals transform the act of making love to a higher purpose. You need to be the type of person who is able to worship your partner as though she were a goddess.

Adopting Tantric Principles

Although most of you probably won't seek out a guru, practicing even the simplest of the tantric techniques can bring a sense of greater communion with your partner, your sexual nature, and, ultimately, with your soul. We become expansive because our spirit opens up when we engage in more trusting sexual practices that involve communication, the spirit of playfulness, and being open to discovery.

Most of us must teach ourselves the basics of love and sexuality through some form of trial-and-error process. Over time, and especially in long-term relationships, we tend to stop exploring and being inventive. When we can break out of those old patterns and learn new ways of being—physically, spiritually, and emotionally—we expand and open. In a sense, we transcend who we thought we were.

Today in the West, there has been a renewal of interest in tantric practices. Perhaps because our society is maturing, or perhaps because of a widespread awakening of consciousness, we seem to be gravitating toward the lessons in conscious intimacy that tantra has to offer. Most of us know very little about our own bodies and our potential for pleasure. In this age of information, we are attracted to what tantra has to teach us about sex and love.

The spiritual seeking that many Westerners are involved in fits well with the practices that tantra offers. The modern seeker may find that many of the components of ancient tantric practices integrate well with our daily lives. In fact, the experiences one has practicing tantra can be seen as a metaphor for other aspects of one's life and can give one tools for being more present and aware in general.

Tantric Sex

In essence, tantric sex is a spiritual practice—like meditation or yoga. It is not meant to be self-indulgent and pleasure is not its only goal. Tantra uses sexuality, with all of its rawness, social stigma, fear, vulnerability, and ignorance to crack open the ego so that we can be present with our lover, and, ultimately, with our self.

FACT

The approximate Sanskrit definition of tantra is web, or that union of opposites that, when united, become one with everything in the universe. Tantric practice aims to unify the many and often apparently contradictory aspects of the self—masculine and feminine, spirit and matter, dark and light—into a harmonious whole.

Sexual Yoga

Tantra is actually a branch in the study of yoga, or practices that help to unify apparent opposites. The practice of hatha yoga, for example, tones the muscles, massages the vital internal organs in our bodies, and contributes to overall good health. It harmonizes the body and the mind by connecting conscious breathing with focusing the mind. When doing yoga, you are actually performing an active meditation. You are focusing your energy on certain internal as well as external points. You bring much more awareness to the body and mind with yoga.

Tantric Gods and Goddesses

Tantra is based on the gods and goddesses of the Hindu pantheon. One telling relationship in this pantheon is between Shiva and Shakti, representations of the male/female, yin/yang energies.

Shiva is the supreme god in Hindu tantra. He represents the male principle and the control and movement of time and all material things. His penis (*lingam* in Sanskrit) is upright, action oriented, and powerful. It commands a place of nerve and worldly power. Shiva's counterpart is Shakti—the female essence. It is Shakti's energy that literally runs the universe. Without Shakti, Shiva is nothing and would have no power in the world. She is the creator, the sustainer, and the destroyer all in one.

These two deities form a union that is necessary to keep the universe in perfect harmony, representing the life of every living human. According to tantric philosophy, life is a journey to become a balanced blend of both male and female, to become whole, or unified. Your sexual nature can lead you to this perfect balance of energies.

Your Guru

The role of the guru in classical tantra is that of guide—a guide who pushes the student to the edge. The guru knows the student and the limitations in that person's life. He sets a path for the student that will ultimately lead the individual to stretch and grow in ways that the student might not attempt on his own.

The beauty of tantra is that it is a partnered path of learning. In a sense, your partner is your guru. To trust another with your personal growth is the ultimate act of surrender, and that's where breakthroughs happen. If two people can do that for each other, taking conscious risks that gently stretch the limits of their comfort zones, they can realize great growth—both individually and as partners.

To risk the vulnerability of doing it wrong, not looking good, being stuck emotionally, and facing your own shadows and life's challenges is to move closer to your own soul and toward the power that resides in self-realization. If you discover, for example, a fear of intimacy and move toward it with courage and trust, without denying it or trying to hide from it, the benefits are great.

Harness the Energies of Your Chakras

In Eastern medicine, the chakras are seven energy centers situated along the spine in what is called the subtle body. Practitioners of Eastern medicine treat the subtle body as well as the gross physical body and see the chakras as very important to the overall health of the individual. Each of the chakras is associated with one of the basic core energies that we work with in life. The energy that flows through them and up the spine is called kundalini energy.

There are symbols, colors, sounds, elements, emotional drives, and gestures associated with each chakra. As you extend your practices of tantra and other teachings relating to the body, you begin to see where you flow and where you get stuck in life. As you learn to sense the energies in your various chakras through tantric practice, you can discover where your life energies are not flowing, where you are stuck, and where you need to put your attention in order to revitalize yourself.

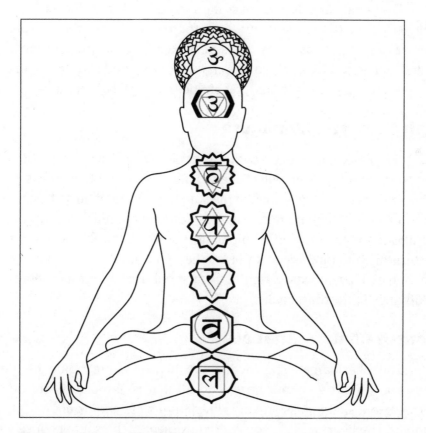

The seven chakras of the body.

The First Chakra: Muladhara

The pelvic area at the perineum is where the first chakra resides. It represents being grounded and secure in the basic physical comforts of life: food, shelter, and the needs of our animal natures. Its element is Earth, and its color is red.

A secure first chakra enables us to feel confident in our abilities to care for ourselves. We can hold a job that brings us enough money to survive. We have a realistic concept of our physical body and its needs and a sense of being grounded.

The Second Chakra: Svadhishthana

The genital area is the seat of the second chakra. It represents our sexual urges and fantasies, creativity, and procreation. Its element is water, and its color is orange. Sensations, pleasure, sexuality, and emotions are all associated with this chakra. When this chakra is open and healthy, we are likely to experience stable emotions, gracefulness, and self-acceptance.

The Third Chakra: Manapura

This chakra is situated at the solar plexus, or navel area, of our body. It represents our power, will, energy, authority, and longevity. Its element is fire, and its color is yellow, like the sun. Ego identity and self-esteem are the products of a healthy third chakra. Confidence, reliability, and autonomy without domination and manipulation produce the fire necessary to live a powerful yet compassionate life. When you have butterflies in your stomach, they may indicate a sign of excitement or fear. This is a temporary disturbance in the third chakra.

The Fourth Chakra: Anahata

The chest area—specifically the heart—is the home of the fourth chakra. It represents our heart and all that is associated with it: sharing, love, service, compassion, and devotion. Its element is air, and its color is green. The heart is often considered the seat of the soul because when it is open it embodies the qualities just mentioned.

We can all recognize the times when our heart feels shut down. This tends to happen when we are mad, hurt, pitying ourselves, or when we don't feel loved. We actually can feel it as a stuck or tight area in the chest. Jealousy has been called the green-eyed monster, and in fact the heart chakra is represented by the color green. We say that our heart aches when we feel the emotions associated with this chakra.

The Fifth Chakra: Vishuddha

This is the throat area of the body. It represents knowledge and speaking the truth of that knowledge. Its element is ether, or space, and its color is violet. The throat chakra builds upon the knowledge learned from the previous four chakras. It takes all that we know and have learned and dares to synthesize and help us speak what we know.

The Sixth Chakra: Ajna

Located at the pineal gland or third-eye area of the forehead, the sixth chakra represents enlightenment and self-realization. It is beyond the elements, so it has no element. Its color is bluish-white. Self-mastery, intuition, and insight are signs of an open sixth chakra. Symbolic and archetypal meaning is integrated into self-reflection. We can move to and through old, recurring patterns in our lives when our sixth chakra is healthy. This chakra often opens up through a spiritual emergence or awakening.

The Seventh Chakra: Sahasrara

This chakra is at the top of the head located at the fontanel, that area where the soft spot is located on a baby's head. It is the open conduit to God and the guru within. Immortality is achieved at this level. It is the realm of saints and of holy men and women throughout the ages. Golden white light and a lotus flower with a thousand petals are the symbols of this uppermost chakra. A supremely conscious human being exhibits compassion, self-awareness, mindfulness, and awareness of the world. Such a person has a highly evolved seventh chakra.

Achieve Tantric Balance

Tantra offers many easy-to-learn practices to help you and your partner evolve spiritually while you enjoy great sex. Many of the practices and lessons in other chapters of this book come from or were inspired by tantric theory, like the repeated reminder to focus your mind on your heart and your partner's heart when you are making love.

Meditation

In many different circles today, meditation is being recognized for its value in bringing focus and quiet to the mind. Its simple techniques are easy to learn and are useful in a variety of ways. As little as twenty minutes a day can bring relaxation, concentration, and lower blood pressure.

At some time or another during sex, most people have found their mind wandering, or have found that they think about whether they are doing it right or about what they wish their partner would do. The highest honor and gift you can give a partner is focused attention. When you bring that quality to your loving, it doesn't matter what techniques you know—you simply *are* a great lover. Practicing meditation will enable you to focus your attention during lovemaking.

Let Your Heart In

Here is a simple practice you can try the next time you are making love. It's about connecting the heart chakra with the genital chakra. Both men and women need to learn to connect the genitals and the heart. Touching these two areas at the same time can bring immense healing, enabling you to experience this connection.

While you are stimulating the genitals of your partner during foreplay or oral sex and, place a hand on her heart chakra. Breathe love deeply into it. Think of the possibility of having a pure heart orgasm or extending the orgasmic release from the genitals up to the heart. You may even want to wave your hand over your lover's body with focus on the heart area. Remind the receiving partner that he can spread the orgasmic feelings all the way up to his heart.

Tantric Orgasm

Tantric philosophy talks about two seemingly different types of orgasm: the physical orgasm and the heart orgasm. At first appearance they may seem contrary to each other, but on closer inspection one supports the other perfectly.

ESSENTIAL

As you go further into this practice, you are able to begin to have full-body orgasms, or energy orgasms, simply by breathing them, without any physical touch. This powerful energy is then much more available to you in your everyday life, sometimes simply by breathing!

Modern sexology recognizes that there are several forms of orgasm. In women there is the clitoral orgasm, which tends to be localized to the genitals. There is the vaginal orgasm, which involves the G-spot and a few other areas of the vagina. There is the blended orgasm, involving the clitoris and the G-spot. Men's orgasms tend to be of one general kind. These are all forms of the physical orgasm. Through tantric practices the orgasmic plateau can be extended for long periods of time. Moreover, tantra offers another kind of orgasm—the energy orgasm, or heart orgasm.

Orgasm from the Heart

Tantric practice encourages us to be in our hearts at all times. That blissful state can be equated to an orgasmic state of being in which heart energy is transferred to all that we experience and do during the day. In tantra this is sometimes referred to as the right-hand path. Certain sects of practitioners achieve this optimum state of being through meditation, yoga, compassionate states of mind, mantra chanting, and celibacy.

In the left-hand path, sexuality is the vehicle one rides to achieve this same blissful state. Sexuality is used as a form of yoga to go to the deepest spiritual levels one can attain. The orgasm is used as the gateway to recognize the bliss state. Once this state of being is recognized, you are able to use that recognition to develop the ability to attain higher states of consciousness that enable you to bring the bliss state to all aspects of life.

When the two paths are blended, the possibilities for personal growth expand exponentially, and the duality between the two types of orgasms vanishes. Just as breath is of the utmost importance in meditation, it is the consciousness of breathing that can be the tool to help you reach a transformational lovemaking experience.

The Kama Sutra

Best known to us for its variety of exotic sexual positions, the *Kama Sutra* has as much to offer modern couples as it did their counterparts in ancient India. Kama means pleasure or sensual desire. It is the name of the Indian god that represents sexual nature in man. Sutra is a short book.

Perhaps the most well known of all love manuals, the *Kama Sutra* was translated from Sanskrit in the mid-1800s by an Englishman named Sir Richard Burton. It shocked Victorian England, and upon Sir Richard's death, his wife burned many of the other books he had translated. Most of them have not been retranslated, and indeed many may be lost to humanity forever.

FACT

The *Kama Sutra*—and anything related to it—continues to be a hot seller. At this writing, a search on Amazon.com for "Kama Sutra" yielded around 7,000 results, ranging from "modern" versions of the Kama Sutra to illustrated guides, videos, and even scented oils.

It is believed that today's known version of the *Kama Sutra* originated from oral traditions passed down in verse form, and that these verses were written and compiled into one book by a man named Vatsyayana. The *Kama Sutra*'s descriptions of the positions are short and to the point. It's almost as if they were meant to be reminders to the couple, rather than detailed instructions. That fact supports the idea that the sutras were born of an oral tradition and were probably originally taught that way to couples.

The Richness of Detail

The variety and depth of information in the book ranges from detailed kissing techniques to seduction and courting suggestions. It explores the idea of biting or scratching your lover to leave your mark on him. Scratching also heightens the sensual feel of the skin during lovemaking. Many different ways of thrusting are mentioned. The positions are named after animals, as this was a prime way of studying man's relationship to the natural world.

ESSENTIAL

The *Kama Sutra* exquisitely describes the quivering of the vagina that usually precedes orgasm and the shuddering that heralds it. It says that no two women make love alike and that one must be very sensitive to rhythms, sentiments, and moods of the individual woman.

Chapter 9 includes some of the kissing and touching techniques from the *Kama Sutra* that have been incorporated into a more modern interpretation. The book describes many different techniques to stimulate the clitoris like the ten types of blows that can be used to tap the clitoris with the penis for stimulation. It details the way in which a man might grasp his penis and churn it from side to side in the vagina of his lover. It outlines what areas in the vagina to stimulate and has special names for the sides, top, deeper areas, and the entrance area.

The *Kama Sutra* also encourages lovers to learn as many of the sixty-four arts as they can, including music, singing, sciences, lovemaking, homemaking, poetry, dance, archery, conversation, sewing, art, games, magic, chemistry, perfumery, and rituals. Refinement and accomplishment were important and were not gender specific.

A Catalog of Aphrodisiacs

In ancient India, the use of aphrodisiacs and their preparation was common and well known to many. Items like datura, honey, ground black pepper, a corpse's winding-sheet, peacock bone, sulfur, pumpkin seed, bamboo shoots, cactus, monkey feces, and ram's testicle were used for enslaving, potency, and endurance.

Some of these ingredients, such as pumpkin seed and datura, are actually well known for their potency-enhancing qualities. However, it may be better for you to stick with some of the more easily procured supplements that are detailed in Chapter 13.

Other Ancient Sex Manuals

Ancient books like the *Kama Sutra* are manuals on lovemaking that were written by people of various cultures for different purposes. For instance, many are guides for newlyweds on kissing, touching, positions in lovemaking, attitudes, moral obligations, and much more. Though Westerners know them to be about positions, these books have a lot more to teach us.

The Ananga-Ranga

The *Ananga-Ranga* was written in the sixteenth century in India. This manual includes morals, seduction techniques, sexual positions, hygiene, rituals and sexual spells, aphrodisiacs, and other erotic concepts. It pays particular attention to the woman learning to control her pelvic floor muscles to heighten the experience between her lover and herself.

The Perfumed Garden

The *Perfumed Garden* was written in Arabia in the sixteenth century. It has a treatise on the many different sizes and shapes of male and female sexual organs. Written primarily for men, the *Perfumed Garden* counsels them to find out from the woman what she likes and ask her for instruction on giving it to her. It speaks highly of God and the gift of pleasure that God has given to humans. It also contains teaching stories of various sorts and many intercourse positions.

The Ishimpo

The *Ishimpo* was a manual that originated in Japan as an erotic teaching manual. Similar to its counterparts in India and other parts of Asia, it depicts the sex act between man and woman as the essential force that controls the universe. It expresses the importance of making love as the force in nature that keeps Earth circling the Heavens.

The Secrets of the Jade Bed Chamber

Exciting many Chinese couples, this treatise on sexuality and sensuality included recipes for potency remedies, exotic positions, and counseling on the ways of love. As with many societies that included eroticism in their cultural heritage, there is symbolism in the words selected for use in the books and by lovers. Metaphors filled the erotic lives of ancient sexual explorers. In the *Secrets of the Jade Bed Chamber*, the penis is described as the *Jade Stalk*; the vagina is called the *Jade Garden*.

Pillow Books

In addition to teaching manuals, China, Japan, and many other Eastern cultures also had pillow books, which were used by couples as erotic stimulants and as reminders of the vast sexual potential any couple could tap into. Beautifully made pillow books were adorned with erotic pictures, poetry, writings, and suggestions that couples could try together to stir their passions.

In the past few decades, there has been a resurgence of erotic manuals, picture books, illustrated instruction books, and a wide variety of resources to educate and reconnect people with their sexual nature. As these materials become available, more people begin to speak openly about sexuality and sensuality. The result is an increasing awareness of our sexual nature and of the variety of touches and pleasurable sensations that turn each of us on.

Positions You Thought You'd Never Try

These ancient books have given us some positions we thought we'd never try. Trying some of them one evening may be just the thing you both need either to get you really involved in new ways to make love or to give you a great deal of laughter all evening long! With names like "donkeys in the third moon of spring," "crab position," and "tortoise position," don't you think you could have a little fun? Here are brief descriptions of a few positions:

- **The Wheelbarrow.** The woman is standing on her hands and has her head on the floor or a pillow. The man is standing, holding the woman's legs. This position is very erotic to the man as he has a bird's-eye view of gorgeous buttocks and the pelvic freedom to thrust effortlessly. It's also known that inversion is quite good for your health, when done in moderation. A variation on this theme is to have the woman resting on a hassock or footstool so that she is a little higher up in relationship to her partner. Make sure the stool won't slip out from under the woman.

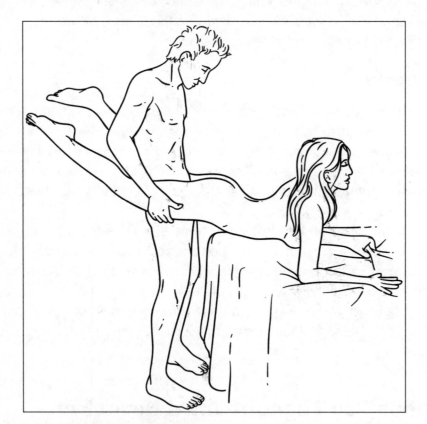

The "wheelbarrow" sex position.

- **Suspended position.** The man stands against a wall or anything that will support his back, and the woman sits on his clasped hands as he holds her up. She is suspended by his arms and holds herself close to him with her own arms around his neck and her legs around his thighs. If she is very small, she can thrust by pushing her feet against the wall that is supporting the man.

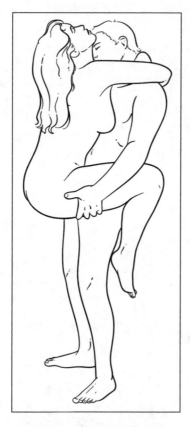

The "suspended" sex position.

- **Three legs position.** Both partners stand together. The woman places one foot between the man's two feet and lifts the other foot and leg so that her lover can hold her leg at the ankle at about the level of his waist.
- **Squatting position.** The man must have very strong, limber leg muscles for this one. He squats and his lover sits astride him, facing him. Her legs are left dangling in the air as he supports her. Subtle movements and rocking achieve the couple's ecstasy.

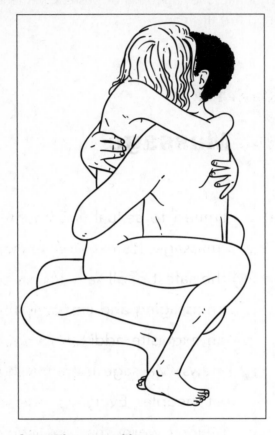

A squatting sex position.

Enjoy trying out these new positions, but be very careful, especially if you think any of these positions may be physically challenging. Endorphins, the chemicals your body produces when you're having fun, can cover up pain.

CHAPTER 15

Sexual Massage

Great sex should never be limited to sexual intercourse. One fun alternative is sexual massage. It's extremely pleasurable, and it's also among the safest of all safe-sex practices. Becoming an expert at massaging and erotically titillating your partner can be an exquisite addition to your sexual repertoire. The good news: Massage is something that comes naturally to most people. Everyone enjoys touching and being touched. Don't worry that you don't know how to do this. Once you start, you'll probably find that your hands and fingers take over and instinctively know what to do.

The Power of Pleasurable Touch

Learning many techniques to give and receive pleasure will benefit you and your partner throughout life. There will be times when intercourse isn't appropriate or when you want to give sustained pleasure to your partner so that he can simply focus on the pleasure without worrying about reciprocating it. Remember that sexual pleasure is a gift. Learning to give exquisite touch during sexual massage will deepen your understanding of your partner and yourself.

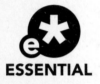

ESSENTIAL

This chapter is written with two partners in mind, but the techniques described here are also very useful for masturbation. The strokes that will be described can help you learn more about your own body. You can let your lover in on your discoveries when the time is right.

Massage Dos and Don'ts

While it's nearly impossible to give a bad massage, there are a few things to keep in mind.

- Do start off with a warm relaxing bath and some soothing music.
- Don't be in a hurry. The whole point of a massage (of any kind) is to relax and unwind.
- Do be gentle, at least at first. If your partner prefers a firmer touch, you can use a stronger grip.
- Don't automatically assume this will be a prelude to intercourse. This may put pressure on your partner. Just enjoy the massage as a sensual and satisfying experience in itself. (Of course, if intercourse does follow, that's a nice bonus!)

Massaging Your Man

During genital massage, find out if your man likes variety, change, and/or innovation. Be willing to ask for feedback and to try new things. Surprise him with some of the techniques in this chapter, then ask him how it feels. When you combine experimentation with focus and loving attention, you will be able to take him to new heights of pleasure. Some of the hand techniques in this chapter are useful for training a man to last longer, too.

Remember that when giving erotic touch, the giver's hands and heart should feel just as good—or even better—than the person receiving the massage. This may sound odd, but if you think about it, it makes perfect sense. We all know when someone is not present with us. We know when the heart is involved to its fullest. Be present with your partner. Focus your attention on how good it feels to give loving touch.

Men tend to like consistent strokes that are typically stronger and harder than women do when they are being touched sexually. They also like variety. Find out just how hard a touch he prefers and just how much variety he would like. Men tend to be very visual, so let your man see what it is that you are doing to him. Prop him up in a comfortable position and let him look.

When stroking his penis, you may have a soft-on or a hard-on to work with. Don't get the idea that one is better than the other. If he seems to be having a hard time relaxing, remind him to breathe deeply into his belly. Rub his belly to bring him into the present and remind him to just lie back and receive. Keep eye contact, when possible, and use lots of lubrication. He'll love the wet, shiny look; and the squishy sounds are erotic.

FACT

Essentials for a sexual massage may include a candle, towels, good-quality oil, and water-soluble lubricant. Relaxing music is also a plus. And, of course, you'll need a warm, quiet area and some love and care to share.

Use your hands, feet, breasts, mouth, hair, fingernails, and anything else that might occur to you when stimulating him. Though we'll focus on hand strokes in this chapter, taking his penis and placing it between your breasts for a few strokes can be a real turn on!

Begin the Massage

Have your clean, relaxed partner lie down. Find a comfortable position that allows you to have both hands free. You may want to start with some light massage to his feet and chest and shoulders as a warm-up. When you are ready to begin massaging his penis, put some lubrication or oil in your hands and gently rub your hands together to warm it.

Begin by gently stroking upward from his scrotum, up over his penis with both hands. Let your hands trail each other so that the motion feels continuous to him, one hand after the other. Move slowly at first and feel *your* hands enjoying the action.

Attention to the Head

Placing one hand firmly around the lower shaft of his penis, take your other hand and begin to gently pull upward with all your fingers on the corona, or the area where the shaft meets the head. This is a very sensitive area, and it loves attention. Pull, tug, and slide your fingertips around and under the head.

In a variation on this, while still holding the lower shaft with one hand, take the index finger and thumb of the other hand and make a ring around the corona. Now twist the two fingers around as far as you can go one way. Let go and make the stroke again and again. Don't move too fast. Ask your partner to coach you on the speed and pressure he likes.

Up and Down

This is the stroke that is the most commonly used by men to masturbate. It's also the one used the most by partners to stimulate the man. Using one hand, stroke the shaft of the penis evenly from the bottom to the head. Use a firm grip and a steady speed. Vary this stroke by putting more pressure on the thumb, either on the upstroke or the downstroke.

Another variation is to stroke just the head this way. You can add variety by doing a few strokes all the way up and down and then a few just over the head or tip of the penis. Then go deep again. You can also turn your hand over and lead downward with the thumb side of the hand, something a man would have trouble doing for himself.

Double Handed Strokes

Using the basic up-and-down stroke, add the other hand to the base of the penis. Hold that hand in place, and use the other hand to do the stroking. The stationary hand can gently squeeze while the other hand is stroking.

Now, with the hand that is stroking, add a twist all the way down to meet the other hand. Twist up and then down. Get as much twist in as you can. Experiment with the pressure. And ask your partner for feedback.

Vary this by using both hands to do the stroking. Try them going the same direction, one after the other, and then try the hands going away from each other and then back together.

Exploring Down Under

Many men like their scrotum gently pulled. This can actually help keep him from ejaculating too quickly. In this move, gently cup his balls with one hand, making a ring around his scrotum with your index finger and your thumb. Pull down. With the other hand, stroke his penis in any way that feels good. You might try a long twist, all the way to the tip and back.

A full one-third of the penis is actually buried under the skin, behind the scrotum. With a liberal amount of lubricant, explore this area. Reach with your hand, under the balls, and gently feel for the root of the penis shaft. With enough lubrication, you can wrap your fingers around the whole shaft. Stroke up and down here while you are also stroking the exposed area of the penis. Men go wild over discovering this hidden area and its virgin nerve endings.

Another area that men often find very erotic is the area just at either side of the base of the penis. This is where the legs meet the torso; many nerve bundles travel through this region. With lubrication, try stroking this area with an up-and-down motion.

You can also stroke and massage the perineum and anus areas while stroking the penis. Many men find this highly sensual and erotic. Some heterosexual men confess that they worry that they might be homosexual after discovering that they like to be touched in these ways. Anal eroticism is not unusual in heterosexual men. These areas have a high nerve count and are very erotic to the touch.

Taking It Higher

Invent some strokes of your own, combining a variety of moves. When you are ready to finish the massage, or if your partner has ejaculated, cup your hand over the penis and scrotum and just rest for a moment. Send your partner love and energy through your hands.

A massage like this can be the tool to learning and teaching ejaculation mastery. Making eye contact, using direct communication, and noticing things like breathing patterns, the two of you can be partners in training him to last for as long as he likes. This may eventually lead him to experience multiple orgasms without ejaculation.

Prostrate, or P-Spot, Massage

The prostate gland and the urethral sponge, or G-spot, are very similar in composition. The prostate pumps the semen out the urethra during ejaculation. If a man is willing and wants to try prostate massage, it is highly recommended. Not only does it feel exquisite, it adds powerfully to the orgasmic sensations and helps keep the prostate gland healthy. While it doesn't take the place of seeing the doctor regularly, a man's partner can keep tabs on the health of his prostate, especially as he ages.

Prostate massage accesses the gland directly through the anus. While some may feel a little squeamish about this, it's not as unpleasant as you might think and the pleasure your partner may derive from it will make up for any initial discomfort you may feel. That said, prostate massage may not be for everyone, so don't push your partner to try it.

Step by Step

If you plan to give a prostate massage, make sure your man is very turned on. Perform oral sex, hand techniques, or any other form of foreplay to really turn your guy on. On a scale of one to ten, he should be at a seven or eight.

Have a latex glove, finger cot, or condom easily available. Use a high-quality lubricant and be generous in the amount you use. Don't use oil; use a water-based lubricant like Astroglide.

With the glove on, spread a liberal amount of lubricant over the area. Tease and play with him a little. Remind him to relax and just enjoy the sensations. Make sure you are continuing to stimulate his penis in whatever manner he likes.

When you feel he might be ready, ask permission to enter him. Use your longest finger. Go very slowly, reminding him to breathe deep into his belly and relax his anal muscles. Notice any changes in breathing, muscle tightness, and arousal. Heighten the stimulation to the penis. Be gentle when your finger is inside him. Move slowly.

Stimulating the Gland

Once inside, reach with your palm up, and feel for the gland. It will feel like a large, soft Life Saver. The center will have a slight, soft indentation, and the round structure should feel firm but somewhat pliable. It will be about the size of a walnut.

Gently explore the sides and center while keeping the stimulation going to the penis. Ask for feedback. As he becomes more turned on, try more pressure. Like the G-spot, the prostate generally can take quite a lot of pressure. Try tapping, rubbing, ringing around the edges, and just holding pressure on the middle indentation.

When you are both finished with this exploration or if he has had an orgasm with ejaculation, don't pull your finger out fast. Ask your partner to take a few deep breaths and as you remind him to relax, slowly bring your finger out. Thank each other for his vulnerability and for your willingness to try this technique.

The first time you try this, you may not get the full erotic feel of it. Keep exploring. After the second or third time, men will really begin to enjoy this massage, but wait a few days before you try it again.

Massaging Your Woman

Women's sexual parts are for the most part hidden, but even so, there are many wonderful techniques that have been pioneered in the past by sexual explorers who have developed strokes and techniques in erotic genital massage for women.

Loving words are like a massage to a person's inner being. Use them when you are giving attention to your woman. Women generally like a much softer touch than men do—especially when it comes to genital touching.

ESSENTIAL

Some women need to learn that it is okay to have pleasure, period. You may find yourself playing an important role—being her guide in the realm of pleasure permission. If such is the case, be generous and compassionate with her.

A woman's vulva and genitals are comprised of mucous membranes that are tender and easily irritated. High-quality lubrication is required in liberal doses. A great guideline for touch is to pretend that there is a bubble of lubricant between the finger of the giver and the surface of her genitals. Then, you can let her know that she can ask for firmer touch when she's ready for it. Some women like consistent moves that continue for quite a while. Other women like to have the touch varied and for change to occur often. Find out what your woman likes.

Remember that, in general, it's less socially acceptable for women to touch themselves throughout their adolescence than it is for men. Your partner may never have explored herself and may need time to discover what works for her and what she likes.

Getting Started

After a relaxing bath, dry your lover with a towel and position her on the bed. She should be lying on a fairly flat surface and shouldn't use too many big pillows—they can keep the body from fully responding to orgasms by collapsing it and blocking the flow of energy. Remind her to breathe deeply into her belly and to relax.

Put some oil on your hands and rub them together briefly. Start with her breasts, and then move on to massaging her belly. Some men have a tendency to use firm touch, but your lover is more likely to respond if you use a light touch.

Apply some more oil and begin to gently brush your hands, one after the other, upward, over her pubic mound. Lightly brush the hair and move slowly. On about the fourth pass over her pubic mound, begin to let your two first fingers delve a little deeper, just over the labia majora, spreading the pubic hair as you do. Repeat these strokes for a while to really build up a charge.

Moving to the Inner Areas

Switch to a good-quality water-based lubricant now (massage oil and interior mucous membranes don't go together very well). Now with both of your hands, gently spread the lips of her vulva. Do this as if you are doing it for the first time—with wonder and awe. Look at her vulva for a moment and tell her how beautiful she is. Begin to lightly touch her inner labia. You can stroke with your fingertips and gently pull on the lips.

With your index and middle finger on either side, stroke from the bottom of her vulva, up, along both sides to the clitoris, and beyond. Repeat this stroke a few times. Now go in the opposite direction. Ask her how that feels. Does she need a firmer touch or a lighter touch? Would she like you to go faster or slower?

Attending to the Clitoris

After you have explored this area thoroughly, move to the clitoral tip. Place your same two fingers above the clitoris and move the hood gently up and down. Now with one hand hold the hood back, away from the clitoris, and with your other hand apply some lubrication.

Begin to explore her clitoris slowly and gently. Move, in very small increments, around the whole outer edge. As you go around, ask your lover what she feels in that particular area. Notice if she reacts more in some areas than in others. Watch for signals her body gives like shifting or slight curling. These may be signs that she needs a lighter touch. Let her know what you are observing.

Once you have located her most sensitive spot, begin small movements in that location. Go in a clockwise direction first; then reverse. See which one she prefers. Now try moving up and down over this exact spot. How is that for her? Stick with the one she likes best for a while and make eye contact whenever you can.

The Clitoral Shaft

Move your two fingers up over the clitoris and place them on both sides. Run your fingers up and down slowly in this area and see if you can detect the clitoral shaft. Now that she is probably more turned on, you may be able to feel it under the skin. It will swell along with the tip of the clitoris.

Continue with this stroke. Bring your fingers close together so that the clitoris is actually slightly squeezed between the two fingers, as you go down over the top. This should be sending some exciting energy to your lover. You might try stroking one side and then the other. One of the sides may be more sensitive than the other because there are more nerve endings there.

If your partner is getting pretty turned on at this point, continue doing the strokes that she likes best. Listen to her responses, both audible and not. Remind her to breathe and relax as she moves deeper into higher levels of arousal. She may want to have an orgasm with just this stimulation or she may want to move on to G-spot massage.

ALERT

Chapter 12 has detailed instructions for finding the G-spot and massaging it. Read this part of the book and refresh your memory if you need to. If your lover is ready and desires to add G-spot stimulation, then proceed.

Massaging the G-Spot

Be sure you are positioned comfortably so that your hands are free. Use one of your hands to continue stroking the clitoris and clitoral shaft. When you think she's ready, ask to enter her vagina with your finger. As you slowly do it, find her G-spot and hold your finger firmly on it for a few moments. Your lover should give you verbal or nonverbal indication that you're on the right area.

Begin to use some of the G-spot strokes you learned in Chapter 12. As you do, time your movements with the movements of your fingers over her clitoral shaft. As you do, be aware that you are stimulating both poles of the woman's sexual parts. As you may remember, the G-spot actually sits between the two legs, or crura, of the clitoris. As the clitoris and clitoral shaft swell with blood, so does the G-spot. These two hot spots are very close together, and as the woman begins to understand and recognize the feelings in this region, she experiences a much fuller sense of her sexual potential.

Continue with this massage for as long as your lover desires. Try the different modalities of strokes and change the pressure you apply to see what she likes. Watch her breathing. Her breath is the key to orgasm and multiple orgasms, so make sure she's breathing deep into her stomach.

Anal Massage

The anal area has many nerve endings and can be a wonderful addition to sexual massage. See if your partner is willing to explore some touch in that area. It doesn't have to mean that she'll be willing to have anal sex later. It just means she is willing to try having more pleasure.

Use a finger cot, a condom, or a latex glove if you'd like. Apply a liberal amount of lubrication. The walls of the anus and vagina are thin. Beyond the very sensitive entrance of the anus, she should be able to feel the G-spot through the wall of the anus. Try massaging her in that area and see. Gently explore.

Continue to massage and stimulate her clitoris as you have been doing. Again, move your fingers in time to each other. Be creative in your dance as a way of showing her that you love giving her attention.

CHAPTER 16

Fun in the Bedroom

Everything you do with regard to your sex life should be fun, but by deliberately making an effort to keep things light-hearted and spontaneous in the bedroom, you can alleviate stress while keeping things sexy at the same time. As you get better at creating new things for you and your partner to experience, your communication and intimacy will increase. Deeper intimacy is a natural byproduct of shared fun.

Sexy Rituals and Traditions

The word ritual may sound formal and intimidating, but when rituals occur in the bedroom they can actually be lots of fun. Anything you do to give an event special meaning or significance (like a birthday celebration) qualifies as a ritual. Rituals and traditions make ordinary occurrences more memorable.

ALERT

Don't confuse a ritual with a rut. Be careful about falling into stale routines simply to take the easy route. If something starts to seem more like a chore than a cherished routine, ditch it and replace it with something new and fun.

A ritual or tradition can be anything you make it. It can be as simple as fixing a candlelit dinner with music and a sensual dessert or as elaborate as creating an entire evening that includes lighting incense, playing special music, toasting each other, erotic dancing or touching, and hours of intense lovemaking. A ritual is designed by you to fit your particular needs and tastes.

The key to creating a ritual is to put your attention on it and your intention in it. You are creating a conscious event that is meant for a purpose. That purpose can be defined, acknowledged, and structured so that it enhances whatever state you want to embody or experience.

Putting It Together

When setting the scene for your romantic ritual, choose the elements that will make for the perfect sensual environment and add some personalized touches that will make this routine uniquely yours. Select colors, scents and sounds that you and/or your partner love.

Consider the purpose of the ceremony. It may be that you have an anniversary coming up, a special day that was a first for you and your partner, or a birthday. Or perhaps you simply wish to celebrate your relationship.

Once you know what your intent is, you can put together your own ritual. Some ideas you may consider:

- Light a candle together as a symbol of your union. A flame is eternal and can serve as a reminder of your everlasting love.
- Share how you feel about your partner, speaking from your heart. This creates an emotional connection between you.
- Music has a powerful impact. Music sets a special tone that, when used wisely, will completely transform and guide an evening. Consider the tone you wish to set: soft and sensual to hot and spicy to holy and serene.
- Incorporate a new sex toy or sensual aid into your ceremony; you can try using a soft fur mitt, a feather, a soft paintbrush, a rose petal, velvet, silk, or sensual foods such as whipped cream.
- Get silly, especially if this isn't normally the way you behave around your partner. What often makes a memorable experience is something out of the norm. Give yourself permission to try things outside the bounds of your usual expression.

Love Ceremony for Valentine's Day

Valentine's Day is the classic time to create a love ceremony. A special dinner, whether at home or at a restaurant, sets the scene for giving gifts and flowers, spending the evening with your partner, and honoring the deep connection and special place you hold in your hearts for each other. The intention is clear and the event is universally recognized. Yet, within this one special day a year, there are many variations to be discovered and created. Here's a Valentine's Day ceremony you can adopt or use as inspiration to create one for yourself.

FACT

Many pagan festivals were reincarnated later as Christian holidays. Valentine's Day originated in early Roman times as a festival of games of sexual license that foretold of the return of spring. It was later Christianized to a day of love and overseen by Saint Valentine, a Christian martyr.

Set aside two hours for the ritual and an additional hour to create the set and setting before the two of you get together. You may need to purchase candles, flowers, fruit (like mango, papaya, small juicy oranges, and kiwi), chocolates, and a sipping liqueur (if you drink alcohol). You may also wish to exchange gifts during the ritual.

Peel, slice, and arrange the food on a plate. This need not be a large amount—you're only tempting the senses of smell and taste, not eating to be full. Pour a small single glass of the liqueur or whatever drink you desire. The two of you will share this glass.

Arrange the bedroom with clean sheets and pillows. Set the candles in several areas of the room that appeal to you. Place one or two candles in the bathroom. Pick soft, sensual music to play. If you've purchased flowers, place them on a table next to the fruit and drink, where you will be able to see them.

When you come together for your evening, tell your partner how excited you are to be having this special time together. Share three specific things that you appreciate about him. At this time, you may also exchange gifts, or you can wait until later.

Take a sensual bath together. Dry each other slowly and accompany your partner to the bed. Exchange massages. Begin without using oils to give a light, fingertip-only massage and gradually explore the subtleties of touch on different areas of the body. Apply a little oil and use a firmer touch, making sure to keep it sensual. The hands giving the touch should be feeling just as exquisite as the body receiving it.

Now face each other, eyes open, and gaze into each other's eyes. Spend a few minutes like this, breathing slowly and deeply into the belly. Gently begin your lovemaking.

There's no rush. Take it slowly and enjoy every moment. Remember to breathe into your belly—full, slow breaths. And remember not to get goal oriented by becoming preoccupied about coming or not coming. Fill your senses with the sight, sound, and smell of your beloved.

Use the food and drink that you've prepared to excite the senses. Tease a little. Ask your partner to close his eyes and let him briefly smell what you are offering first. Lightly brush the morsel across his lips, allowing him to feel the fruit's texture.

Weave and dance through your lovemaking. Speak to your beloved. Be vulnerable and open, even if it's not that easy for you to do. Remember that your lover wants to hear what you are feeling. Tell your partner how much you appreciate his love. Let him know how precious this time is to you.

Sensual Food Fun

Playing with your food takes on a whole new meaning in the sensual and sexual context. The possibilities are almost endless when you consider how many foods are considered either sensual in their texture and appearance or actually have aphrodisiac properties. Whipped cream and chocolate sauce in bed is just the beginning.

Create a sensual meal that is made up of finger foods. Include textures that are sensual to the mouth and lips. Place the food in a beautiful setting—why not recline over pillows strewn on the floor? Make a rule: Neither one of you can feed yourself, but you can feed each other!

There are good books available on this subject. Try Diana De Luca's *Botanica Erotica* for more fun ideas. She includes body butter recipes, erotic drinks, a guide to erotic herbs, and a variety of food ideas in addition to recipes for making your own tinctures.

ALERT

Sugar is one of the worst things you can put into a vagina. Anything with even a slight amount of sugar in it can cause immediate reactions and can lead to a yeast infection in the woman, and possibly in the man. Be extra careful when playing with food applied to the body.

Intimate Games

Simple games can have a unique place in intimate relationships. They can be fun and challenging. Some people will take to them a little more easily than others. Know your partner and, if you are going to introduce the idea of games into your love-play, pick ones that will be fun for both of you.

Games can teach you new things about your partner. They can gently push boundaries and open new realms. And they can open up a Pandora's box full of dark secrets, perceived danger, and adventure. Mostly, though, they are fun and a good cause for humor and lightheartedness. They introduce a new approach to sexuality that we don't often come up with ourselves, and they can be cause for opening up the imagination for creation of your own fun and games.

It's important to remember to respect your partner at all times. If something isn't working for one of you, the game is over. Many love games involve surrender and receiving. It is difficult for some people to completely receive from the other. This is something that can be learned. Here are a few ideas to get the juices flowing.

Take Away One of Your Senses

Sight is a powerful sense—perhaps the strongest of all our senses. It is the first sense we draw on in everyday life. It is a powerful driver of experience. When we take it away, we give much more control to our other senses.

Play a lover's game that will help you heighten your senses and increase your awareness of touch and sensation. As part of an evening of experimental fun, you can create a game around the sense of touch without the sense of sight. Design an evening of exploratory fun that will also train the two of you to pay attention to your other senses.

Find a rose, a piece of very soft fur, a new art-style paintbrush, a feather, or anything that will produce a very sensual feel. You might even want to have a few ice cubes handy. Have a soft scent in a misting bottle and a gentle bell or chime handy. Gather at least four items. Set the scene by lighting candles, putting on soft erotic music, and having something to nibble (strawberries, a little chocolate, or some mango pieces will do!) and something to drink close by. Blindfold your lover. Now use your imagination.

Swimming in Oil

You can also create a fun game using warmed olive oil. To play, set the scene and the mood by lighting candles and making sure the room is warm. Throw some towels or an old rug that you don't mind staining on the floor. Prepare extra towels and something to drink and nibble on. Gently heat 2 to 3 cups of olive oil in a saucepan. You can add a few drops of a pure essential oil for fragrance if you wish.

When you are ready to begin, both of you should shower. If you have long hair, you may want to pull it back. Put on your favorite erotic music. As you are sitting on the towels, begin to apply olive oil generously to each other's bodies. Go ahead and really get into it. You're going to get very oily!

As you oil each other, you'll notice an incredible freedom to slip and slide all over each other's bodies. Enjoy this sensual experience to the maximum. You'll feel as though you've never had so much of your body touched and stimulated at one time. Be playful. Fun is the name of the game here.

If you want to move on to making love, you need to clean off the oil first; salad oil may not be your lubricant of choice.

Pulp Fiction

Write your own pulp fiction. Each of you can write an account of your ideal erotic fantasy, then read these aloud to each other. This is a great turn on and a wonderful exercise in spontaneous self-expression. Get pens and paper, and just write. Don't think. Just write for ten minutes. Or pick another erotic subject that you have thought of ahead of time. Take turns coming up with the subject. Examples: "The best orgasm I ever had" or "The riskiest sex I ever had." Read these to each other.

Or you can use an intimate apparel catalog as a starting place for an intimate story. Have either the models in the catalog or you two be the subjects. Create an erotic adventure tale.

Be Creative

As you move from games to lovemaking, be creative—don't just opt for the same few positions in bed. If you've got some privacy, explore the rest of your house. The kitchen table is often the perfect height for intercourse. Try the counter for oral sex. Have the woman bend over the arm of the over-stuffed chair in the living room for rear entry. The women can also sit on the arm of the sofa and have her partner kneel on the cushions as he enters her. This is a good position in which to put one of your feet up on the back of the couch. Choose the side of the couch that will best allow you freedom of movement and maximum G-spot access.

The most important point here is that you should feel free to be creative and experiment. Take turns thinking up new places and ways to make love. You've nothing to lose and a whole lot of fun to gain!

Get yourselves a hassock—they are fantastic for a modified yab-yum position (see Chapter 10). The man sits on the hassock and his partner sits on top of him and closes her legs around him. He supports her back with his hands. This position is easy on the man's back. It gives both partners the freedom to rock, grind, and undulate to their hearts' content.

Another option is to forget furniture altogether and spread a lush carpet or blanket in front of the fireplace. Bring as many pillows out as you can find, to give you a variety of options for shaping your environment to suit the positions you might want to try.

Take It Outside

The ancient Kama Sutra texts talk about the physical health and psychological growth that can become available to you when you break away from your normal habits of lovemaking. When you move into nature, for example, you can mimic the birds and the bees, the lioness and her suitor, or two fishes swimming side by side. Being outdoors can add an element of mystery and erotic excitement to the sex act. You can become more aware of yourself and your partner when you remove yourselves from your usual surroundings.

It's often difficult, in modern living situations, to get to an outdoor place that feels safe for expressing sexual love. If you have a backyard that is private, you can create specially landscaped areas that may be conducive to lovemaking. Or try a gliding porch swing, a piece of lawn furniture, or a love-swing in different places around the yard or in the house. All these things will add titillating new variations to your lovemaking.

You may be inspired by the wild sexuality displayed in mating rituals of different animals. Go to the zoo with your partner or look at nature videos. Check out how the animals do it. In many ancient societies, it was believed that animals can teach and inspire us in our own lovemaking.

Go out into nature and observe, and get inspiration for new positions. Swim like the fishes and try undulating together underwater. Use your nails to scratch lightly and your mouth to bite gently. Use sound to add to the variety. Growl and howl, groan and whimper, moan and hum!

CHAPTER 17

Relationship Stresses

Even the best relationships involve stress. Confrontation, heated discussions, spirited debates—these are all present in healthy relationships. No matter how much of a perfect match you and your partner are, you will inevitably have disagreements, differences of opinion, and even the occasional passionate argument. Then there are outside stresses: work, family, and money. And, of course, many couples experience stress related to their sexual relationship.

What You Can Expect

Power struggles—and the stress that accompanies them—are a fact of intimate life. This doesn't mean your relationship is on the rocks or that your partner has suddenly turned into an arrogant jerk. Every relationship, even those that may look perfect from the outside, has its share of stress, conflict, and emotionally charged disagreements.

So what can you realistically expect?

- You will be disappointed.
- Your feelings will change.
- You won't meet each other's every need.
- You will learn how to forgive.

You Will Be Disappointed

That's the bad news. The good news is that, with a little luck and a lot of work, you'll learn not to take these disappointments personally.

Intimate couples will inevitably encounter disappointment. When you know to expect this, when you know it does not mean the beginning of the end, then you are more empowered to take disappointments in stride. You can communicate your hurt feelings to your partner and hear her response. You can discuss how you each experienced the incident in question. You can acknowledge that it was not your intent to hurt or disappoint, or that you wish you had not promised more than you could deliver. Then you can forgive and begin again—and again!

Your Feelings Will Change over Time

When you meet someone you find attractive, at first you will pay more attention to the positive, attractive aspects of that person. Even if you notice faults or foibles that you don't like, these will most likely take a backseat to the qualities you appreciate. This stage, which may be called the romantic stage, is just the first of five that most relationships go through as they mature. The other four are power struggle, stability, commitment, and cocreation.

It Begins with Romance

Romance is the stage in which we focus on our similarities and the things we like about each other. It is the stage in which we go out of our way to be pleasing. This allows a bond of trust to form, and we often feel that "here is a someone who will love me as I am; I can feel safe with this person."

Although this stage eventually passes, you can recall how it made you feel and bring some of those feelings back into the present. To help you reconnect with the essence of romance, recall what first attracted you to your partner. Take a few minutes to remember how you felt when you two were first falling in love. If you have never discussed this, or if you have not discussed it lately, make this a topic of conversation within a few days. It can help to rekindle some of those young-love feelings.

As you reflect on that romantic getting-to-know-you period, you might also notice that some of the things that first attracted you have now changed. This fact could lead to disappointment, unless you can remember that change is to be expected. It's a necessary part of the journey. What most people do not realize is that once a strong trust bond is established in a relationship, partners tend to feel safe enough to reveal themselves and their negative aspects more fully.

If things have changed for the worse, it's not because your partner was intentionally deceptive. It's more likely due to the fact that once a romantic bonding occurs, your partner feels safe and secure enough to be more open around you. This leads to the next stage, power struggle.

ESSENTIAL

Intimacy doesn't just happen. It takes time, effort, and communication for a couple to become truly intimate with each other. While the romance stage is great, you won't achieve real intimacy until the later stages of your relationship.

Power Struggle

During the romance stage, two people may seem like the perfect couple. Their sex drives may be in sync, and they think everything the other one does is cute and funny. Then time goes by, and things may change. Their sex life becomes less exciting (perhaps even nearly nonexistent). They don't seem to be connecting anymore.

ESSENTIAL

> You know you're in the power struggle stage when you try to get your partner to change so that you can feel better. Stop and ask yourself why you feel you absolutely need those changes to occur. Can you love your partner for who she is?

If anything like this has ever happened to you, remember that what you get to see of another person during the romance stage is like the tip of an iceberg. When you first meet someone, you cannot know this person all at once. You can't yet see what's hiding beneath the deep, dark waters—the other 85 percent of the iceberg that will be revealed over time.

The power struggle stage is the stage during which formerly hidden differences in wants, needs, and expectations rise to the surface. Power struggles can be resolved if you and your partner are able to recognize that these struggles may originate in unfinished emotional business from your past. To get beyond such struggles and heal any unresolved issues, you must enter the stability stage.

A Time of Stability

As your relationship goes from the power struggle stage to the stability stage, you learn that the outer struggle mirrors the inner struggle—that is, if your partner's behavior triggers intense anger or hurt, this probably indicates an area where you have unresolved emotional issues within yourself.

Stability is the toughest stage to master. For most people, a partner can be a ready scapegoat. It's so easy to blame someone else for your pain—all he'd have to do is change one little thing and then you'd feel better! When you let go of blaming your partner, even secretly, and take responsibility for your own emotional triggers, then you are solidly in the stability stage.

From Stability to Commitment

If you succeed in mastering the lessons of the stability stage, the rewards are great. In the commitment stage, you can enjoy a genuine sense of safety—not the illusory safety of romance. Now you really feel your unity, your interdependence. You become a we, where you naturally consider how your actions will affect your partner.

Such thoughtfulness comes, not from any sense of obligation, but from a deep knowing of and empathy for the other. But you need to go through the other three stages together before you can arrive at true commitment. Now your promises to each other are trustworthy. They were not before because you had not yet met and mastered the basic life task of taking responsibility for yourself (the task of the stability stage). Until you pass beyond stability, you are still secretly or not so secretly looking to be taken care of, as in, "I want you to stop flirting with other women because it makes me feel insecure." (Translation: It triggers my insecurity.)

Cocreation

Once two people are aligned in their oneness and secure about their ability to make and keep agreements without any sense of obligation, they can create things together with a real sense of partnership. They might create simple things like nice dinner parties for their friends. They might coauthor articles or teach classes together. Or they might use their bond to support each partner's individual self-expression in the world.

Cocreation is where you reap the rewards of the work you have done in the other four stages, and where you give back to the world from what life has taught you. The couple's journey from romance to cocreation helps both partners learn to be comfortable with change. It can help you avoid needless disappointment over the fact that "you're not the person I first fell in love with."

You Won't Meet Your Partner's Every Need

Even when you're first falling in love, you are probably aware, in theory, of the fact that you will not meet your partner's every need. Theory is one thing, but hearing your partner say they want to go somewhere with a special friend instead of with you—well, that might not be so easy to accept. Has this happened to you? If it has not, be prepared, for it probably will.

If it never happens, your relationship is not very mature. You're probably still babying each other or the relationship, treating it as too fragile to handle such conflicts. In any relationship, there will be things one partner wants to do that do not include the other person. If you try to avoid mentioning such things to avoid causing discomfort, then you will not progress very far in your journey as a couple.

Sure, it can hurt to hear your partner say that she would rather be with someone else, or alone, than with you. It hurts, but it's good for you, in the sense that by facing the truth—that you do not meet each other's every need—you also grow in your ability to handle life as it is.

Learning to Accept Differences

Here is an exercise to try with your partner:

1. First, each of you should make your own list of all the things you love to do.
2. In the left-hand column next to each item, write A (for things you prefer to do alone), Y (for things you prefer to do with your partner), and O (for things you like to do best with someone other than your partner).
3. Now share your lists and talk about your feelings. As you share feelings, be sure and start with the words "I feel." Using these statements will prevent you from attacking, blaming, or judging your partner.

After doing this exercise, give yourselves credit for taking on the challenge of being honest about difficult things. Being honest about your needs for separate space will bring you to a deeper level of intimacy and trust—trust that is no longer seen in terms of "I trust you to never hurt me" (which is unrealistic), but rather in the following way: "I trust myself to be able to handle whatever feelings come up between us. I trust that if you do something that hurts me, I will talk with you about it. And I trust that you and I together can listen to each other's feelings nondefensively so we can get to forgiveness." This is a real, mature relationship.

You Will Learn to Forgive

Forgiveness is an essential survival skill in any relationship. No matter how mature and responsible two people become, they will do dumb or hurtful things at times. Forgiveness can occur in an instant. But more often it is a process that takes place over time.

Usually there are several elements or stages in the forgiveness process:

- Figuring out what happened.
- Investigating what you feel.
- Expressing what you feel to your partner.
- Listening to your partner.
- Expressing other feelings.
- Forgiving each other.

Beware of premature forgiveness. Many people cannot stand the discomfort of anger or resentment, so they say "I forgive you" before they have even found out what happened or fully explored their feelings about it. To get to true and lasting forgiveness, you need to be willing to go through all the stages until you feel a change of heart within yourself.

What Happened?

The first step in any forgiveness process is to identify what your partner did that resulted in anger or hurt feelings on your part. You need to think clearly here, because people are often hurt by something they imagine or by their interpretation of their partner's actions.

Ask yourself, "What really happened? What did my partner actually do or say?" Then ask, "What happened after that? What was my reaction? What did I actually feel? What did I say or do about those feelings?"

What Do You Feel?

After identifying what you felt after it happened, notice what you feel right now. Are you still upset? Are you feeling pain or hurt feelings? Notice the actual feelings and bodily sensations and do not be confused by your labels and judgments. "I feel betrayed" is actually not a feeling. It is an interpretation about the other's actions—you think someone has betrayed you.

If you are thinking, "I do feel betrayed," see if you can pinpoint the exact feelings that you associate with betrayal. Getting upset can trigger old feelings—feelings that happened long ago but were never fully admitted or expressed and so were never released. So now, when a similar feeling occurs, you may mistake it for that same old wound. You overreact in the present to an experience that appears similar to some unresolved hurt in your past.

Expressing What You Feel

For most people, this step is the hardest of all. You may fear that your partner will be defensive or maybe that you'll create a mess. But if you take that risk now, you won't have to carry the burden of your unexpressed hurt and anger all by yourself. And you probably will get over it once you talk about it with your partner. Remember—the purpose of expressing your feelings is to get over them, to get to forgiveness.

Listening to Your Partner

After your partner has heard you out, listen to him express his own feelings and perceptions. Ask clarifying questions to help your partner be more specific, but don't put him on the witness stand. Questions that begin with "Isn't it true that you . . ." are forbidden.

As you listen to your partner, it's a good idea to use active listening. Repeating what your partner has just said keeps you grounded and present and prevents you from reacting impulsively. It also helps your partner feel that you are present and open, thus increasing the likelihood of resolution.

Expressing More Feelings

Now check in and see if you need to express anything more. Sometimes simply stating your resentments clearly, specifically, and directly leads to a sense of forgiveness: "I'm over it now. . . . I can forgive you. . . . I just needed to express myself and be heard."

Other times, you may still feel almost as upset as you did when you began, so you will need to repeat yourself. Simply restate what you said before; if you become aware of some new feelings, express them as well. After each expression, check in with yourself to see if you feel clear yet. Do you have a sense of resolution or closure?

Keep expressing yourself, even if you think it sounds repetitive, until you feel complete. Sometimes, the process of expressing strong anger will result in a surfacing of fear or pain. Sometimes anger will surface after you express hurt or painful feelings. Do not be alarmed if you discover something hidden underneath your initial feelings.

ESSENTIAL

Sometimes, to get to a feeling of completion, you may need to repeat these steps together a few more times. If a present hurt is similar to one that you suffered in the past, the wound may not heal all at once. Be patient. Accept that emotional wounds, just like physical ones, can take time to heal.

The human psyche is like an onion with many layers. Once you express yourself fully about a particular incident, feelings about another event might come into your awareness. Sometimes, you will be reminded by the current situation of something that happened to you long ago, maybe when you were a child. If this happens, then be sure to tell your partner that old buried feelings are now coming up. This allows your partner to be a compassionate listener. Then ask your partner to bear with you, and just keep expressing yourself.

Forgiving Your Partner

Once you feel complete in your expression, you are probably ready to forgive. It helps if you can truly realize that your triggers were set off by your partner's actions. Your partner is not to blame for that. Your partner is responsible for her actions, but no one is to blame for what you experienced.

You need to remember that blame is not real. It is a defensive reaction that people use to feel more in control about something that happened. It is more mature to admit that you do not have control over things done by another person. The blaming habit supports an unrealistic view of reality—a view that says, "If I hurt, it's someone else's fault." Pain happens. The best way to deal with life's painful moments is to feel the pain, talk about it, forgive, and continue living.

CHAPTER 18

A Lifetime of Sex

Great sex is something you can enjoy all of your life. You are never too old to enjoy a satisfying sex life. In fact, as you get older and more mature, you often develop skills that allow you to become a better lover. Each partner and relationship you have adds to your library of sexual knowledge, as does any research or studying you do (such as reading this book). If you have the desire to keep learning and improving, you can have great sex that lasts a lifetime.

The Very First Time

When you feel secure, empowered, and self-confident, most things you do for the first time will go well. Having information, knowledge, and resources helps you have even better life experiences. This is definitely true when it comes to your first sexual experience. Whatever your age, you need to remember that sex can happen with or without intimacy, love, and commitment. Sex may be a part of a young person's explorations of who they are. It can be the result of giving in to the peer pressure of keeping up with friends. It can be a way of testing both how lovemaking might feel and how or who one is in relation to gender and sex.

Don't Rush In

Generally, parents, clergy, and educators all feel that teenagers and young adults should put off sexual activity until they are more mature. However, young people who feel like adults and are out to test their boundaries and experience life don't often follow that advice. It might be helpful for them to know that many people who have sex for the first time at an early age later realize they weren't totally ready for the experience and wish they had waited.

ALERT

If you are a parent of a teenager who is interested in sex, sometimes all you can do is trust that you have done a good job of educating your child and hope he or she will make wise decisions because of that. If you have younger children, make sure you take an active role in educating them about sex.

If you are a teenager and think that you're ready for your first sexual experience and you would like it to be healthy and fulfilling the first time, there are several things you may want to consider. Make sure you have spoken with your potential partner and that you both agree that you're ready to be together; ideally, you will also be able to speak with a parent or another trusted adult in your life, especially if you have any fears or frustrations. It's also important that you have a safe, comfortable place to be with your partner.

Many young people don't know much about sexuality. Have an open conversation with your potential lover. Chances are, this is a first for him as well, and you may discover that both of you share some of the same fears.

Your first sexual experience is something you'll remember for the rest of your life. Try to make it the best possible. It will get you started in the right direction on the road of sexual growth that will take you through the rest of your life.

Talking to Kids about Sex

As a parent, it is necessary to have safe, open conversations with your children about many things in their lives: drugs, alcohol, peer pressure—and, of course, sex. You won't be able to talk about sex easily with your child unless you like it yourself and have already had other conversations with them about important things in their lives. Start talking to them now so that you can do it later when it's really important. Here is what you need to keep in mind as you begin:

- Sex education isn't a replacement for parental advice. Don't leave the sex talk up to the school. The information and advice will be more meaningful coming from you. Besides, teachers are often restricted by school policies and state laws as to what exactly they can include in a sex ed curriculum.

- Start early. If you wait until you think your child is considering having sex, you may already be too late. Today, more than two-thirds of eighteen-year-olds have already had sexual intercourse.

- Always be on the lookout for teachable moments. Don't lecture—ask your child what he thinks about something presented on TV or in a magazine. Construct your questions to be nonjudgmental so that your child feels permission to speak up. The conversation will last longer that way.

- Teach equality and self-esteem to your child. The current thinking among teens is that oral sex isn't sex. It's a very popular activity, and it allows girls to claim they are still virgins. Most of the oral sex is performed on the male, not on the female. This sets up a girl-pleasing-boy scenario and an early imbalance in sexuality and intimacy. It perpetuates the cultural permissiveness of sexuality for boys and the double standard of "innocence of body" for girls.

Protect Your Children

Here's a scary statistic: estimates are that one in four girls and one in six boys will be sexually abused before age eighteen. The most shocking part is that the perpetrator is often someone the child knows and trusts. Small children need advocates. It is often impossible for them to be able to judge what is appropriate and what is inappropriate behavior from a trusted adult. You can educate them in nonfearful ways, such as by teaching them the difference between "good touching" (such as a hug or a handshake) and "bad touching" or by viewing a "stranger danger" book or DVD that is age appropriate. You can be watchful over the children in your life. It is very appropriate for any adult who suspects child abuse to talk about it with other adults. Don't just watch from the sidelines—if you suspect abuse, do something about it.

Making Love with a New Partner

Chances are, you have had a few sexual partners in your life. Some of these relationships may have been more casual than others. The more special your partner was to you, the more shyness, fear, or even guilt you may have felt the first time you had a sexual experience with this person.

ESSENTIAL

For both young and old, being naked in front of your partner for the first time may be very frightening or it may be erotically charged—or both! If you anticipate having a new lover, take it slowly and express that you are feeling vulnerable. It may help to undress each other.

When you are just starting out a new relationship, you may feel pressured to impress your new partner sexually, and you may want to do it better than in the past. You ask yourself if you really did learn anything from your mistakes and struggles from your previous experiences. You can use the communication, intimacy, and touch techniques covered in this book to get to know your partner intimately in a fun, relaxed manner, before you decide to take the next step toward sex.

The "Highs" of a New Relationship

Many people are addicted to the "rush" they get from a new relationship. When you begin a new relationship, the endorphins often take over and cloud your vision for a while. You feel on top of the world and the relationship feels indestructible.

Eventually, though, you'll come back down to Earth. It's then, as the relationship continues for the long term, that you will need the tools to help you stay clear and loving. If you take things slowly and build your intimacy skills and connection in the new relationship, it will go well. You will both be able to sustain those highs that attracted you to each other in the first place.

A Beginner's Mind

Even if you are in a long-term relationship, you may find it helpful to have a beginner's mind—being open, vulnerable, and trusting in your sexuality. A beginner's mind isn't full of judgments or complaints about how you want things to be. It accepts things as they are and works to transform both the interior struggles and the behaviors that lead to problems.

Sexually Transmitted Diseases (STDs)

Sexually transmitted diseases (STDs) are very prevalent today—and have been throughout history. Though we have good prevention methods and effective treatments, STDs remain a growing concern among doctors, young adults, parents, and sexually active adults.

What Are STDs?

As the name implies, STDs are viruses, diseases, and other medical conditions that can be spread via sexual contact (although many of them can also be spread via other means).

How Are STDs Spread?

Sexually transmitted diseases are contracted through the following forms of sexual contact:

- Genitals (including the anus) to genitals
- Mouth to genitals
- Genitals to hands to genitals
- Mouth to mouth (only for some STDs)

Treatment of STDs

STDs may be caused by bacteria or viruses. The bacterial forms are generally treated with strong antibiotics. The viral forms cannot be cured, although their symptoms can be treated with antiviral drugs.

Common Sexually Transmitted Diseases

Except for HIV, the viral infection that causes AIDS, all common STDs have plagued humans for thousands of years. The symptoms are more noticeable in men. Women are more likely to have STDs that go undiagnosed; they can be unwitting carriers of the disease.

Here are descriptions of common sexually transmitted diseases that you should be aware of. Chlamydia, syphilis, and gonorrhea are bacterial infections; the rest are viral.

- **Chlamydia.** This STD is very common and hard to detect. Three-quarters of women have no symptoms. Symptoms can include discharge, burning, and pain during intercourse.
- **Syphilis.** This chronic disease is acquired from someone with an active infection. The first signs are painless sores that go away easily; long-term effects include damage to the heart, brain, eyes, bones, nervous system, and joints.
- **Gonorrhea.** There are often no symptoms associated with gonorrhea. When symptoms do appear, they may be mild but can include discharge from the penis, vagina, or rectum, and burning and itching during urination. There is an alarming increase in gonorrhea of the throat in teens who perform fellatio on their partners.

- **Human papilloma virus (HPV).** Genital or venereal warts is the most common STD in the United States. It is very contagious and is becoming associated with cancers of the genital regions. The warts are fleshy growths in the genital regions; they do not cause pain.
- **Genital herpes.** The symptoms of this virus include itching, burning, and blisters in the genital area or buttocks. The open sores are painful and the lymph nodes can become swollen in the groin area.
- **Hepatitis B.** This virus is acquired by piercing the skin with needles and through exposure to semen, blood, saliva, and urine from an infected person. Most infections clear up, but if they aren't, the liver can be affected. In extreme cases, hepatitis B can be deadly.
- **HIV/AIDS.** The human immunodeficiency virus develops into AIDS after the virus has destroyed the immune system and left the person vulnerable to infections. To date, there is no cure.

The AIDS Epidemic

With the AIDS epidemic sweeping the world, greater knowledge and preparation is needed. In an age when pleasure can quite literally kill, education, open discussion of sexuality, and easy availability of preventative resources must become the norm. Here are the main ways HIV is transmitted:

- Anal or vaginal intercourse with an infected person
- Oral-genital sexual activity with an infected person
- Contact with semen or vaginal fluids of an infected person
- Organ transplants or blood transfusion from an infected person
- Contact with infected blood through the use of contaminated needles from drug users or tattooing, ear piercing, or steroid injections
- Transfer from mother to child during gestation, birth, or soon after birth (breastfeeding is risky for an HIV-positive mother)

FACT

The most typical fluids through which HIV is transmitted are blood, semen, and vaginal secretions. It has been documented to be present in urine, saliva, tears, and feces, but there is no evidence of anyone contracting the disease through any of those avenues.

When to Seek Help

People are often embarrassed to seek help if they think they might be infected with an STD. No matter how nervous or embarrassed you may be, it's important to seek treatment. In many cases, your symptoms can be eliminated or reduced through medications or other treatments. Your doctor can also tell you how to avoid spreading the STD to your partner(s).

Practice Safe Sex

If you are going to be sexually active, make sure that you're protected! People who have multiple sex partners have a higher risk of contracting STDs, and people who start sexual activity at a young age are also more likely to have STDs. Don't be afraid to ask your potential new lover about his sexual history, and be willing to talk about your sexual history as well. Your lives may depend on it.

See your doctor frequently. If you have any question in your mind, get tested. If you don't want to go to your regular doctor, you can go to a number of clinics where you can be tested anonymously.

Being a Conscientious Lover

Having good self-esteem and a conscientious attitude are both very important when discussing personal sexual histories with a new partner. The accepted method of clearing yourself and a new partner for unprotected sexual activity is to be tested at the time you decide to take your relationship to a deeper level. While you wait for your test results, you can begin to share intimate experiences that do not involve intercourse or other risky behaviors.

Knowing a lot about sensual and sexual touching techniques can help when you are with a new partner. The previous chapters have many techniques to choose from. You can begin to get to know each other's bodies until the time you decide to take the next step to intercourse. Of course, you have the option of using condoms, too.

Latex, Condoms, and Finger Cots

Condoms made of latex are the safest method, outside of abstinence, for staying disease-free. By preventing direct contact between the penis and the female sexual organs, condoms protect both the man and the woman from contracting sexually transmitted diseases. They can prevent pregnancy by keeping the male ejaculate from entering the vagina, but they are not failsafe.

There are also female condoms, though some women say they can bump the cervix and are slightly uncomfortable. That may change as new products are introduced to the marketplace in the next few years. Dental dams are square pieces of latex that can be used to cover the female's genitals for oral sex. Plastic wrap can be used, too. Finger cots, or condoms for a single finger, are good for anal stimulation and erotic touch over the genital areas.

All of these items provide a good barrier against the transmission of sexually exchanged diseases. Don't hesitate to use them. They can even add fun to the experience. If you are having sex in a situation that warrants protection, make it fun and worry-free for both of you.

Responsibility

Many women say they feel it is ultimately up to them to make sure they are having safe sex. They say it is important to be prepared and to not be talked out of using male or female condoms if they feel it is warranted. This can be difficult if you have self-esteem issues that might keep you from defending your boundaries.

Sex During Pregnancy

Most doctors agree that unless there are medical complications during a pregnancy, there is no reason a couple cannot have normal sexual relations. Your doctor may not broach the subject with you, but you can bring it up if you have questions. Your own intuition should serve as a good guideline for sexual activity.

Typically, by the third trimester a woman may have difficulty with some sexual activities because her uterus becomes distended. During intercourse, her cervix may get bumped, causing slight pain. Her changing hormone levels may also make her less interested in sex.

Most couples find other ways to enjoy each other. Use some of the suggestions in this book to invent new ways the two of you can pleasure each other during pregnancy. It's a great time to practice oral sex and other forms of sexual activity.

Finally, this will be the last time for a while that the two of you are just two—particularly if this is your first child. Find ways of being sexual, sensual, and intimate now, even if you have to modify what you do. Traditionally, doctors advised women to refrain from sex for six weeks after childbirth, but today many doctors advise abstaining for at least two or three weeks. Obviously, this varies by individual circumstances – if you have medical issues or experienced problems during the delivery, you may need to wait longer. Sleep, time, and energy will be harder to come by, but most couples fully resume sexual activity after six to twelve months.

Sexuality and Aging

It's challenging to adapt to changing hormones and body agility and accept the changes our bodies go through as we age. Today, we have many options for staying perpetually young in looks, health, and spirit, so middle age isn't so daunting on the surface. When it comes to sexual vitality, though, things do change as your body ages.

Health Issues

The good news is, we're living longer and you'll want to have sex longer as well. The bad news is that as a culture we are more overweight, more dependent on prescription drugs, and have higher incidences of cancer. These cancers are prevalent in the areas of the body that have to do with sex. Cases of breast cancer, testicular cancer, prostate cancer, and uterine cancer are all on the rise.

Maintaining a healthful lifestyle is very important for great sex. Eat well, stay fit, and see your doctor regularly. Educate yourself on matters concerning health and sexuality so that you will be well informed when aging issues come up.

Maintaining Sexual Desire

Desire can be elusive throughout your life. Many people experience ups and downs in their level of desire. Depression, stress, and anxiety all contribute to lowered levels of the brain chemicals that keep us optimistic, healthy, and full of desire.

Lowered hormone levels during pregnancy, illnesses, and personal crises can cause the loss of sexual desire. Midlife menopause in both men and women can cause confusion about desire and desirability. Many modern medications and drugs used for depression and stress-related illnesses can cause a complete lack of libido.

Lifestyle issues also affect the quality of sex as you move through different periods of your life. Very often, after women have had their children, they go back to work with a vengeance. They put in long hours and come home to more hours of creating and maintaining a sanctuary in their home. They may be absolutely enjoying themselves, but it does make for a long, exhausting day.

At the same time, they are gently aging. Their testosterone and estrogen levels are dropping. Estrogens regulate the monthly cycle and help stabilize the emotions, side effects, and physical sensations of menopause. Testosterone gives women energy and sexual vitality the same way it does for men, although women need a much smaller amount of the hormone than men do.

Men's testosterone levels drop as they age, too. Their desire may begin to wane, though it may be attributed more to performance anxiety and fears associated with declining libido and perceived sexiness. Men seem to be much less willing to address the issues.

Training Your Mind

Desire has a lot to do with how you've trained your mind to think about sex and sexual attraction. If you have been sex-positive for most of your life, it's likely you'll be more sexually active as you age. If you find that you encounter problems, you will be more likely to seek out remedies and solutions for them.

Our brain is our biggest sexual organ. We can enable ourselves to feel sexy, stimulated, and desirable by training our brains. It's never too late to start. Sex and desire are healthy, normal functions of any human being. If you or your partner is concerned about the lack of desire and libido, consult your doctor and ask for a referral to a sexologist.

Dealing with Menopause

If you are a woman who has reached (or is about to reach) menopause, you may be distressed by the changes in your life, including some negative effects on your sex life. Luckily, there's a lot more you can do to alleviate your experience of menopause. Here are a few suggestions:

- Physical activity is key to leading a healthy lifestyle. Find an exercise program that you enjoy and make it a part of your everyday schedule.
- Avoid stress. Take more personal time for yourself and cut back your work hours.
- Create sensual (but not necessarily sexual) time with your lover. Be playful and innocent—it doesn't have to go anywhere as long as you enjoy touch, massage, and cuddling.
- Practice your PC muscle exercises. Being proficient at these will bring more blood flow to your pelvic floor area, keep you toned, and will actually help build your sexual energy and sexual desire.
- Try estrogen and testosterone topical creams. These will stimulate your libido and heighten sensation in your erogenous zones.
- Attend a sexuality or tantra workshop with your partner. Workshops can put a tremendous amount of new sensual energy into relationships.
- Consider taking up yoga and meditation. These activities teach you to focus your attention and keep your body supple. Focusing techniques can help you respond better to the sexual stimulus that you receive.
- Don't be afraid to use lubrication, if needed. It can be erotic and fun to apply. There are many products on the market already, and new lines are appearing that are organic and natural.
- Keep a sense of play and innocence when introducing new experiences. And most important, have fun!

Get yourself a good book on menopause; one good option is *The Everything® Health Guide to Menopause*. It will give you all the information you need to understand what is happening to your body, mind, and soul.

CHAPTER 19

A Do-It-Yourself Sex Workshop

Now it's time to put together everything you've read about in this book so you and your partner can enjoy a lifetime of great sex together. This chapter will present six specific sexual self-help programs: four are for couples, one is for partners who are just beginning a sexual relationship, and is one for people who wish to prepare themselves for great sex with a new partner.

Adding New Spices to an Old Recipe

If you are fortunate enough to have been with your partner for many years, it may be time to spice up your sexual and romantic life. Perhaps you have gotten into a routine that is comfortable but lacks excitement. Perhaps you have begun to avoid sex entirely due to a backlog of incomplete communications. Perhaps there are still things that are frustrating or difficult, even after all these years. Perhaps you feel the need for variety but don't want to go outside the relationship for it. If any of these issues speak to you, read on!

Breaking the Routine

It takes conscious effort to get out of your rut, but the effort is well worth the time it takes. If both of you have read this book, it's now time to have a conversation with your partner about which ideas for adding spice and variety appeal to each of you.

In Chapter 16, you learned about many ways to make the place where you make love more sensual and beautiful by using colors, flowers, and fragrances, and by bathing each other, feeding each other sensual foods, and dressing erotically. Some of these ideas may bring up feelings of fear or embarrassment, but you need to go beyond these initial feelings—all of these suggestions may be just the thing for spicing up your sex life.

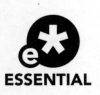

ESSENTIAL

Your partner can be your greatest ally and healer! Don't give up too easily. A recent study found that married people had far lower rates of depression than people who are not married. Choose to do the intimacy work that will make both of you overflow with happiness.

If you do something that feels a little scary, it means you are taking a risk on behalf of the relationship. You are stretching your comfort zone, and your relationship is growing. You may have heard the saying *grow or die*. This means that if you're not stretching in a relationship, your relationship is dying. Don't let your sex life die an untimely death. Keep it alive and fresh by consciously changing things every so often.

Getting Back in Touch

No matter how long you have been together, you never outgrow your need for touch. Being touched in sensual, sexual, and nurturing ways helps people feel relaxed, loving, and loveable. Chapter 9 presents a wide range of touch exercises to revive your senses and renew your capacity for whole-body pleasure.

If you two have been together a long time, you probably have not had a "how I like it served" conversation recently—what feels good to you during foreplay and beyond—which is something that couples need to address often. Just because things are working fine, it doesn't mean that you should fall into complacency.

Sometimes people's needs change over time. Sometimes, as you get more comfortable with yourself or your body, you learn new things about yourself. Don't let yourselves get out of touch with each other; keep communicating and trying new things.

If Variety Is the Missing Spice

There are many ways to add variety to an already satisfying relationship. Try a new position. Do it outdoors or on the kitchen floor. Try one-way sex in order to give each person the chance to simply receive pleasure. Try having sex without orgasm for a month.

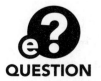

QUESTION

I need a shift from the routine. What can I do?
Imagine a weekend away at a luxury hotel, a camping trip, a cabin in the mountains, or a seaside resort. Pick a place were there isn't much to do except stay in your wonderful hideout. Take along a Kama Sutra kit, massage oil, scarves, a love game, lingerie, champagne, or anything else you can come up with!

If you have not explored the G-spot or the anal area, see what that holds for you. Dress up as someone different and act out the part (maybe you still have that old cheerleader outfit stored away somewhere). Have a fight about something you've both been avoiding. All these things can renew your feelings of love and lust. Try any of them that appeal to you, or better yet, try them all.

Connecting with Her Sexual Essence

It has been said that if sex works for the woman, it works for the man. Many of the tantric and other ancient practices described in this book offer ways that allow the woman's response to guide the way for both partners.

Foreplay Revisited: Don't Rush It

If the woman is not enjoying sex as much as you both would like, the first place to look to remedy that situation is foreplay. The same old foreplay routine can often feel boring for the man. But if that's what she likes, it will behoove you to learn to tune in to her needs rather than viewing it as simply servicing her.

When two people feel connected, when they are tuned in to each other, boredom disappears. A woman can help her man tune in to her by giving him verbal and nonverbal feedback about how he's doing. Most men report that they'd like a lot more feedback from their partner about what feels good.

Moaning and making other sounds are one good way to do this. Chapter 11 recommends using breath and sound—both as a way to help your partner know where you are and as a way to enhance your own responsiveness.

Communicating Wants

Many women are shy about asking for what they want. If this is true in your partnership, it's good to talk about this outside the bedroom. First talk about her fears—what she's afraid will happen if she were more expressive. Then talk about what she wants. It's the old "feel the fear, and do it anyway" principle. Fear is a fact of life. Don't let it limit you too much.

If the man wishes to help the woman express herself more freely, he can use some of the communication practices from Chapters 4 and 17. One of the techniques that helps a lot is to give her a multiple-choice question to answer, such as, "Would you rather have me do this with more pressure or less?" With this type of question, a woman who is afraid of hurting the man's ego, or even one who doesn't know what she wants, can be helped to accept and reveal her preferences.

Trying New Positions

The position that works best for the man is often not the woman's favorite position, and vice versa, so please don't allow yourselves to gravitate to the man's favorite if he happens to be the one who is clearer about his wants.

This may cause the woman to yield in ways that are not in the best interests of great mutual sex. So, even if you have gotten into a pretty good routine together, don't assume that things could not get even better. Keep experimenting with new positions.

Enhancing His Pleasure

Sometimes it is the man who needs more help enjoying sex. Because of the fact that a man's self-esteem is often closely tied to his sexual performance, he may be reluctant to admit that things could be better for him. Yes, men fake sexual interest just like women do—they just do it differently.

To reduce the likelihood of pretending, withholding, or faking, partners need to help each other feel safe admitting when things aren't feeling quite right. Give your partner permission to tell the truth about what he wants. Don't take his self-disclosures as criticism of you.

Men Need Warming Up, Too

Somewhere in high school many men got programmed to believe that they should always be ready—just in case the opportunity ever comes along! But as they mature and as sex gets to be more available and less of an opportunity, this attitude becomes inappropriate. A man should not expect himself to always be ready whenever the woman wants it.

This being the case, a woman needs to learn to feel comfortable with a limp penis. Do not wait for your man to be hard before you touch him or put your mouth on him. And pleasure his whole body, not just his sexual parts. This book offers a wealth of ideas for getting both of you in the mood.

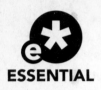

Letting his lover be active in lovemaking is healing for the man. It helps him outgrow his conditioning to be always active and in charge. It helps him learn to let go of needing to run the show and discover that he is loveable even when he is not doing anything to earn love.

Passive and Active

Most women are conditioned to be passive. Don't deprive your man of the pleasure of feeling your hunger for him. Just because you were conditioned to act a certain way, it doesn't mean you have to stay that way. If you think you'd like to learn to be more active in sex, a good way to start is by giving your man a full-body massage that culminates in an erotic massage, as described in Chapter 15.

Sex after Sixty (and Well Beyond)

Sixty is not so old anymore. People are taking better care of themselves and living longer. Many men and women older than age sixty have sex that is just as satisfying as it was when they were younger. However, they usually do it less frequently.

Letting Go of What Used to Be

Some people feel sad when they notice their sex drive growing less intense. Others celebrate this fact. If you are in the former category, the secret to making this transition successful is to allow yourself to experience your feelings of sadness and loss fully.

It's also important to be honest and transparent with your partner about such feelings. Let's say, for example, that your partner doesn't reach orgasm as easily as before. How do you feel about this? Do you feel afraid? If so, what meaning are you giving to this fact that creates the fear? Or maybe you feel angry. Again, what are you telling yourself about what this change means?

If you imagine that it means something significant, be willing to check out your assumption. Ask, "I notice you didn't come the last few times we've made love. I'm afraid that means you're no longer interested in sex. Is that true?"

Less Busyness Equals More Bliss

Sex after sixty can be better than it was in earlier years because you may now have more time to enjoy it without as many distractions. If you are no longer working at a regular job and are no longer responsible for kids, you have a lot more free time to explore the subtler aspects of sexuality.

Throughout this book, we have emphasized the importance of simply being present in each moment. When your lifestyle is less pressured, you may have more chances to fully experience the moment-to-moment nuances of sexual sensations, including how your sensations are influenced by your breathing and by where you put your attention.

Feelings of love, conscious breathing, and paying attention to your bodily sensations are still the best aphrodisiacs there are. These things can continue to develop over an entire lifetime. They are not limited by age.

No Erections Necessary

Tantric sex teachers encourage men and women to become as comfortable with a soft-on as they are with a hard-on. Lots of pleasure can be achieved by rubbing your two bodies and pelvic areas together. Many people find this a wonderful alternative to penetration—especially if the woman's vaginal tissue has become thin or sensitive.

A soft-on can also be inserted into the lubricated vagina. From there, experiment with various movements to see how they feel. If this feels good to the woman and she lets him know it, it will often start feeling good to the man as well. If you are willing to accept what is and work with what you have, rather than focusing on what you don't have or can't do, you will continue to discover new realms of pleasure well into your later years.

Oral sex is fabulous when your man has a soft-on. There's less urgency, softer tissue, and more time to play. You may have the experience of having him grow in your mouth—and then again, you may not. Simply enjoy the experience without any expectation.

You're Never Too Old for Erotic Touch

Even if you have little or no desire for intercourse, you still need to be touched in a loving way. If sexual intercourse does come to a halt, don't stop teasing, touching, kneading, and stroking your partner's whole body, including the genitals. You never outgrow your need for touch.

Beginning Things Right

A new sexual relationship may be fun and exciting, but that's no reason to get complacent. Now is the very best time to explore conscious lovemaking and expand your capacity to experience pleasure.

Communicating Expectations

Talk to your new lover about what having sex means for your relationship. What are your expectations of each other? Does having sex carry hidden expectations or hidden fears?

If you have secret questions or fears about this topic, or secret expectations that you aren't aware of, this conversation will help clear the air so you can be more present to each other during lovemaking. If you leave these sorts of things unaddressed, you'll be thinking about them when you'd rather be enjoying your newly found love.

Sex Lessons

The second conversation that needs to occur should examine what each one of you likes. What turns you on? What secret longings do you harbor? What fetishes and fantasies do you have but are reluctant to disclose?

A good way to have this conversation is to do part of it as a show and tell. While in a relaxed, tender mood, allow your partner to see what you do to turn yourself on. Let her move your hand to the spots that give you most pleasure. Let your partner play with you as you give feedback on what feels good, better, and best. It's often fun to give your preferences numbers, like, "That's a ten . . . that's a seven . . . that's only about a two," and so on.

Read this book together, perhaps taking turns reading chapters to each other. Then discuss anything you think you might want to try. Talk about any feelings or shyness that comes up. And have fun.

Creating a Romantic Mood and Setting

Make your first sexual experiences special by creating a romantic setting for lovemaking. Delegate one of you to set the stage, preparing a special atmosphere that honors both partners.

ESSENTIAL

Simply sitting together very closely and gazing into each other's eyes for five or ten minutes is an experience of bonding, trusting, presence, and relaxation. It's a great thing to do on one of your first dates with a potential new partner. You'll both learn a lot from the unspoken.

Leave lots of time for sensual exploration and foreplay. Do not rush it. If your lives are too busy, plan some time away from your normal routine. And definitely turn off your phones and avoid other distractions. It's important that your early sexual experiences leave time for lots of trial-and-error learning. That way you will not fall into habits that need to be corrected later.

Time to Bond

The early stage of a relationship is a time for sexual bonding. Busy people often do not take the time to bond properly. This takes more time than you might think.

Bonding occurs when two people share unstructured tender time together, both inside and outside the bedroom. So if your love is new, spend a day in bed together now and then, talking, cuddling, resting in each other's arms, and, of course, pleasuring each other and getting to know each other's bodies.

Getting Yourself Ready for Love

If you do not have a sexual partner, reading this book and doing the exercises will help you get ready to have one. People say that chance favors the prepared mind. You have a better chance of attracting a great sexual relationship if you have prepared yourself with the necessary knowledge and skill.

Are You Ready?

Is anyone ever fully ready to love and be loved without reservation, without fear? Probably not. So if you don't feel completely ready, don't make too big a deal out of this. The truth is, practice makes perfect.

There is someone out there for you right now—someone who could love you just as you are. There could be many possible reasons you have not connected with this person, and some of these are beyond your control. However, one thing is in your control: your degree of preparation. You can, for example, keep sexually fit even if you do not have a partner. You can use every social situation as an opportunity to hone your communication skills. You can do whatever you can to heal your unresolved issues from the past. And you can get clear about what you truly want in a sexual relationship.

How's Your Sexual Fitness?

It's important to stay healthy and fit, whether you're in a relationship or not. Do not neglect this aspect of life just because you don't have a partner at the moment. If you let this go, you will be less attractive to potential partners. Health and sexual vitality are a turn on. You will feel more attractive and alive when you have a positive relationship with your own body.

Healing from Past Wounds

Perhaps you do not feel ready to begin a new relationship due to unresolved conflicts from your past. Maybe you have felt betrayed or have simply been disappointed too often. If this is the case, it's good to recognize that your next relationship may not be the love of your life. You are probably not ready for that. You may need to have a learning relationship or a healing relationship first.

In seeking such a relationship, start by being honest with yourself that you want someone with whom you can be yourself and who will not expect you to be anyone other than who you are. This means he will not demand a commitment from you. You may find someone with similar needs. You can admit that you're not ready for a full-on commitment and look for someone to share what you do have to offer.

CHAPTER 20

Your Health and
Its Effects on Sex

Emotions and chemistry play a big role in a good sex life. But, let's face it, sex is a physical act involving your body and its assorted parts. And if your body isn't feeling 100 percent, your sex life will probably suffer. Even if the desire is there, your health and medical issues can make it difficult for you to enjoy sex to the fullest. Of course, some health issues may be out of your control. But by taking good care of yourself, practicing healthy habits, and taking all possible steps to minimize any health problems you already have, you have the best chance of enjoying a satisfying sex life.

How Your Health Affects Your Sex Life

Your health affects your sex life in many ways. For one thing, it's tough to be enthusiastic about doing anything when you don't feel so great. Also, sex—at least in most cases—requires physical strength, endurance, stamina, and other traits that can be compromised by health problems.

Good health is also important to fuel your desire and interest in sex. A healthy body produces sufficient amounts of hormones to keep your sex drive at maximum levels.

You probably already know that good health allows you to feel more physically fit and strong. This is very important for any type of physical activity, including sex. Can you imagine how disappointing it would be if you were just starting to engage in some passionate lovemaking with your partner, but had to cut things short because you were too weak or tired to continue?

Physical issues also have a tendency to blend into mental and emotional areas, as well. If you are worried or stressed about your health, you may not be as emotionally supportive with your partner as you should be, which will in turn impact your sex life. It's all connected.

Conditions That Often Cause Sexual Problems

There are many health conditions that can wreak havoc in your sex life. Some of these may be obvious. If you're having urological issues, for example, or if you're a woman with hormonal imbalances or conditions involving the uterus, ovaries, or anything in that region, you probably wouldn't be surprised to discover that your sex life may suffer, at least a little bit. On the other hand, you might be caught off guard by the sudden decline in your sex life as a result of seemingly unrelated medical conditions.

Diabetes

It's not unusual for men with diabetes to suffer from impotence, at least on an occasional basis. Diabetes can negatively affect blood flow to the penis, making it difficult for a man to achieve and maintain an erection as often as he may like. In addition, the fluctuations in energy levels through-out the day (especially if your diabetes isn't well controlled or you don't follow your treatment plan) can affect sexual interest and stamina for people of either gender.

High Blood Pressure

High blood pressure causes a problem similar to the one caused by diabetes. Damaged and/or hardened arteries and blood vessels carry less blood to vital organs and appendages, including the penis. Plus, high blood pressure can cause headaches and other symptoms that generally don't put you in the mood for romance.

FACT

Although medical conditions involving reduced blood flow have the biggest impact on the physical sexual abilities of men, women are not totally off the hook. Reduced blood flow to the genital area in women can cause vaginal dryness and discomfort. Fortunately, lubricating gels can be very helpful in solving this problem.

In what can seem like a catch-22, the medications commonly used to treat high blood pressure are also notorious for causing sexual problems. See more details in the section on medications.

Heart Problems

Heart problems and circulatory issues often go hand-in-hand. Again, there's the issue of poor blood flow to the genitals.

Then there's the fact that people with heart conditions can often find it more difficult to do any kind of strenuous physical activity. Unless your heart condition is very serious, it's likely that sex is safe for you (but of course you should check with your doctor to make sure). If you find it painful or exhausting to over-exert yourself, you can simply avoid the more acrobatic positions and focus on sex positions and techniques that you find both enjoyable and physically comfortable.

People who have already had a heart attack or heart surgery may be especially nervous about having sex, even if their equipment seems to be working fine. While you will likely need to refrain from physical exertion of any kind for a certain period, most patients can usually resume normal sexual activities after a short time, once their doctors give them the okay.

ALERT

Because erectile dysfunction can be caused by an underlying medical condition, it can sometimes alert you to a serious health problem you didn't even know you had. This is yet another reason why it's important to discuss the problem with your doctor.

Multiple Sclerosis

A large number of people with multiple sclerosis experience some form of sexual dysfunction, ranging from erectile dysfunction and premature ejaculation to decreased sensation in genital areas. MS can sometimes cause painful muscle cramps and spasms that make sex impossible or painful.

Depression

Many people suffering from depression will have little or no desire for sex. This really isn't all that surprising—especially in the case of moderate to severe depression, where people often have little interest or motivation to do anything enjoyable at all. People who are depressed also tend to want to be alone, which of course isn't exactly conducive to having sex.

Hormonal Disorders

Hormonal imbalances and disorders can cause sexual problems in both men and women. Generally, this appears in the form of low sex drive (or no sex drive at all).

According to the National Institutes of Health, about 5 million American men have low testosterone. In addition to impotence and other sex problems, low testosterone levels can cause breast enlargement, hot flashes, and depression.

For men, low testosterone levels frequently cause erectile dysfunction and other sexual problems. Low testosterone can be caused by aging, accidents, testicular cancer, and other health problems.

Excessively high testosterone levels won't be so great for your sex life, either. Too much testosterone in men can cause aggression, acne, and other nasty side effects.

Testosterone levels fluctuate throughout the day, often following a somewhat regular pattern (for example, many men have higher testosterone levels in the morning). If you or your partner are alert enough to track these patterns, you may be able to tailor your sexual routine so you can take advantage of those peak testosterone periods.

Testosterone isn't just an issue for men. Women who have too much testosterone will often have manly traits such as excessive facial and body hair, increased muscle mass, and deeper voices.

ALERT

Anabolic steroids cause many health problems, but are perhaps most notorious for causing impotence and other sexual problems in men. This is because steroids cause testicular shrinkage, which leads to performance problems along with low sperm count and infertility. There's also a strong tendency toward aggression and rage, which of course doesn't encourage warm and intimate relations.

Many women are distressed to suddenly experience sexual problems during or after menopause. This is caused by a drop in estrogen levels. While hormone replacement therapies can help, they carry their own side effects and risks, so talk to your doctor and research all your options before deciding what's best for you.

Conditions Affecting the Pituitary Gland

The pituitary gland is a small gland attached to your brain. It secretes hormones and controls other hormone-releasing glands, such as the adrenal glands. That means this gland has a lot of power over your sex drive. Unfortunately, that also means that any problem with your pituitary gland—such as a tumor (even a noncancerous one) or a cyst—can really wreak havoc with your sex life.

Many people know that thyroid problems can affect weight and energy levels. However, you might be surprised to learn that thyroid imbalances and conditions can also cause low sex drives and impotence.

The Good News

If you have one or more of the health conditions that have the potential to adversely affect your sex life, you may be feeling a bit nervous, even if your sex life is going just fine at the moment. Don't despair—there are lots of steps you can take to keep your sex life going, regardless of your health issues.

These include:

- **Erectile dysfunction (ED) treatments.** If you suffer from ED, there are several medications that are effective in treating this condition for many men. You must of course first tell your doctor about any other medications you take, to avoid any negative interactions.
- **Libido boosters.** If your sex drive isn't what it used to be, you may just need to jump start it. Try watching some adult movies or engaging in new forms of foreplay.
- **Oils and lubricants.** For medical conditions that cause vaginal dryness, use lubricants or oils. You don't need to focus on the remedy aspect, because these products can enhance your sexual experience and are great for everyone, whether they have dryness issues or not.
- **Energy boosters.** If health issues have sapped your stamina, try a few different energy boosters (protein shakes, multivitamins, etc.) and see if you notice any improvement. Ask your doctor for suggestions of products that can help your energy level.

Medicines and Sexual Side Effects

While prescription medications can be an important part of your medical treatment plan, they can also sometimes have annoying or unpleasant side effects. There are numerous medications that are known to cause sex-related side effects.

Diuretics

Diuretics, commonly known as water pills, are prescribed for a number of conditions that can cause water retention, including high blood pressure and heart problems. They have been known to cause erectile dysfunction in some men.

Beta Blockers

Beta blockers are commonly prescribed for high blood pressure and heart conditions. They can be a lifesaver for many people, but for some men these drugs can also lead to erectile dysfunction.

Antidepressants

Many traditional depression medications have been linked to erectile dysfunction and decreased sex drive in both men and women. However, some of the newer antidepressants are said to be less likely to cause these types of side effects.

Speak Up

If you do experience any kind of sexual problems—especially if the problems started suddenly and coincided with a medical problem or a medication you started taking recently—it's important to discuss this with your doctor. Many people are reluctant and embarrassed to mention sexual issues to their doctors, but in many cases your doctor may be able to recommend an effective solution. Often, it's as simple as switching to a different medication. There's no reason for you to suffer through a bad or nonexistent sex life when a simple chat with your doctor can lead to a solution.

If you are hesitant to discuss your sexual problems with your doctor, think of your partner. Remember, you aren't the only one being affected by this problem. Your bedroom issues also affect your partner, probably in a big way. So if you can't do it for yourself, do it for your partner. In the end, you will both reap the benefits.

How Your Sex Life Affects Your Health

Now that you know how your health affects your sex life, consider the flip-side. How does your sex life affect your health?

Many studies and articles have touted the health benefits of a good sex life. It's believed that good sex can help lower blood pressure (once the frenetic bedroom activity is done, of course), alleviate depression and other mood disorders, and just make you healthier and more energetic overall.

An active sex life gets your blood pumping and works out your muscles. It burns calories and motivates you to stay active and work up a sweat in other ways, too.

A rewarding and satisfying sex life also puts you in a more positive and happy frame of mind, which in turn makes you more likely to take care of yourself. Plus, a good attitude can make a big difference when it comes to the state of your health. And if you and your partner are enjoying a satisfying relationship with a good intimate connection, it's more likely that you will support each other's healthy decisions and take care of each other.

A Healthier, More Sexual You

The good news about the sex-health connection is that there are many steps you can take to improve both your health and your sex life at the same time.

Become Healthier Together

For one thing, you can make your healthy lifestyle a joint activity. Recruit your significant other to be your health and fitness partner. Perhaps the two of you can get into the habit of working out together—or, if you are the athletic types, playing tennis or another activity. The rigorous physical activity will get your blood pumping, and the adrenaline rush may help put you in the mood for sex. Many couples find it sexy to see each other all hot and sweaty.

If you aren't quite that athletic, perhaps you can take long walks together in the evening. This offers some added perks: It allows you to unwind from a stressful day and lets you enjoy some quality time together and share important conversations.

Don't Forget Your Diet

While exercise is a major component in a healthy lifestyle, a sensible diet is equally important. You and your partner might find indulgent dinners to be romantic, but they may not be helping your waistline. Of course, an occasional dietary splurge is fine, but the majority of your meals should be relatively nutritious. Don't worry; nutritious doesn't need to be bland or boring. There are plenty of cookbooks and TV cooking shows devoted to healthy-yet-tasty meals. Make this a joint activity by planning healthy meals together, and enjoy some quality time together while you shop for the perfect ingredients.

Encourage Each Other to Stay Healthy

If you or partner has any health issues or concerns, it will affect both of you in the long run. Make sure your partner knows how important her health is to you, and remember that the feeling is probably mutual. When your partner is worried about your health, she will be anxious and distracted—and this will surely put a cramp in your romantic life.

Provide moral support for your partner and encourage her to seek help for any medical issues or concerns right away. On the flip side, alleviate your partner's concerns by doing the same thing whenever you have health issues of your own.

ESSENTIAL

If your partner is reluctant to seek medical advice or treatment for a health problem, you might need to give her the guilt treatment by telling her how worried and stressed you are about it, and how relieved you would be if she took action. Then remind her of all the things the two of you plan to do together in the future—plans that could be in jeopardy if health problems get in the way.

A Good Health Checklist

Staying healthy can seem like a big job, but you can boil the main priorities down to a few important (and, for the most part, relatively easy) steps. Let's review some of the key things you can do to stay in tip-top sexual condition:

- Have regular sex.
- Eat a diet rich in whole grains, high-quality proteins, fresh fruits, and vegetables.
- Do your Kegels.
- Do regular aerobic exercise.
- Manage your stress; balance play and work.
- Be moderate in your eating and your alcohol consumption.
- Don't smoke.
- Get regular checkups and practice good preventative care.
- Seek treatment for any medical issues as soon as possible.
- Don't engage in risky behavior.

CHAPTER 21

Modern Twists

Like everything else, sex has taken on some modern twists in the twenty-first century. True, the basics are still pretty much the same: You and your partner are still using the same body parts your ancestors used and are essentially performing the same biological act that people have done throughout all of history. But there are some new toys and other extras that can give your sex life an exciting modern spin.

Cybersex

When you think modern, you probably also think high-tech. And perhaps the most obvious modern sex tactic is cybersex. This is sex or some sort of sexual activity that involves a computer. Cybersex has gotten somewhat of a bad rap, because it is often used in underhanded ways, such as when someone wants to secretly engage in sexual exchanges with someone besides his or her partner.

However, when used by a couple to enhance their sex life, cybersex can be fun and exciting. Cybersex can take different forms. It can mean having virtual sex with your partner, with each of you at a different computer. Couples often engage in cybersex when one partner is out of town, say on a business trip, but they still want to share a sexy and intimate experience. Or you can even engage in some cybersex while both of you are at home, on computers in different rooms. This can be a fresh and exciting form of foreplay.

How It Is Done

Engaging in cybersex doesn't require a lot of technical expertise. You each need a computer and some way to communicate on a real-time basis. Usually this involves instant messaging, which allows you to communicate back and forth with instant responses. However, it's also possible to have an online sex chat via e-mail.

If you each have a headset or microphone, you can speak to each other while sending your online messages. Another benefit of cybersex: You can add images (either of yourself or of anything or anyone sexy you find online) to your messages, to add some visual stimulation for your partner. If you are familiar with using online video, you can even include a racy video clip. When you put all of these visual and audio elements together, it's like taking old-fashioned phone sex and adding some exciting new bonuses.

Variations

While cybersex in itself can be pretty exciting, there are ways to take it to an even more thrilling level. Here are a few ideas:

- You can each create virtual characters of yourselves. Feel free to enhance certain physical attributes to match your partner's fantasy. Then use your headsets to supply the vocal soundtrack as your online personas enjoy some racy encounters.
- Begin your online rendezvous when one or both of you are in a public place—say, at a business meeting or in the airport. See how exciting it is to tease your partner when they are forced to maintain their composure. For your partner, it will heighten the anticipation. He will be counting the minutes until he can go somewhere private and fully enjoy the second half of your cybersex session.

Cybersex with Someone Else

Another option is engaging in cybersex with someone besides your partner. You should only do this if your partner is okay with it. You both need to be in agreement as to whether cybersex is real sex, in the context of fidelity. There's a big debate about this, and many people do consider it cheating if their partner has cybersex with someone else. If you do decide to try this, only do it when your partner is present and aware of your activities. Doing it behind his back will indeed seem like you are cheating.

The great thing about online communication is that nobody knows anything about your appearance, personality, or other characteristics except for what you tell them. If you've always wanted to be taller, thinner, more muscular, more outgoing, or whatever, this is your chance. Don't feel guilty—most likely, the other person isn't exactly as he describes, either.

ALERT

If you engage in cybersex with a stranger, you should use common sense and take safety precautions. Never use your real name or reveal any personal details about yourself. And if the other person says or does anything that makes you nervous, log off and cease communication immediately.

Your partner may find it a turn-on to watch and/or listen while you engage in cybersex with someone else. This can actually be a relatively safe variation of the sex with a stranger while your partner watches scenario that some people find exciting. Unlike with real-world sex-with-stranger encounters, there's no need to worry about your partner's history or health status.

Here's one sexy approach to cybersex with a stranger: When you and your partner are in different locations, make a date to log on to an adult chat site at a pre-arranged time. You should each keep your own user names or online IDs a secret from your partner. Then proposition someone from the group and engage in some sexy banter. How explicit or hardcore you get is up to you. The illicit thrill here is that you won't know if you are having cybersex with your partner or a stranger.

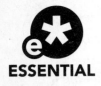

ESSENTIAL

If you do engage in any type of cybersex with someone besides your partner, be alert for any clues that you may be chatting with someone who isn't an adult. Teenagers posing as adults often like to use these sites. If you have any suspicion that you are dealing with someone who isn't of legal age, cease all communication immediately.

Online Porn

Pornography was covered briefly in Chapter 12, but there is a specific kind of pornography that has increased in popularity in the past few years: online pornography. As the name implies, this is pornographic material that you view on the computer or another electronic device, like a cell phone that has web access. You can find online porn very easily, simply by doing an online search using whatever specific keywords relate to your particular sexual preferences or tastes. And you can be sure that no matter how unusual or strange your tastes and fetishes may be, you can find plenty of adult online material that will fit the bill.

According to statistics compiled by TopTenReviews.com in 2006, more than 42 percent of Internet users visit porn sites, more than 25 percent of all online searches are porn-related and around 10 percent of adults admit to having an online porn addiction. Their statistics also show that 70 percent of women keep their online porn activities secret.

Advantages of Online Porn

Online pornography offers many benefits over traditional print pornography. For one thing, online porn is easily accessible. You can get it simply by sitting at your computer. There's no need to leave your house. An added bonus: You don't have to summon up the courage to venture into the adult section of your local newsstand or bookstore. And you don't need to endure your mailman's smirks when you receive a package in that telltale brown wrapper.

Since you view online porn in the privacy of your own home, it's more discreet than other forms of pornography. There is also an incredible amount of variety when it comes to online porn. No matter what your particular preference or fetish, you are sure to find plenty of online porn that turns you on.

In addition, you can access quite a bit of online porn for free. However, watch out for unexpected charges.

ALERT

Resist the temptation to check out online porn at work. Even just a quick peek can land you in a lot of hot water. Many companies now routinely monitor employees' online activities. Even if you use a company laptop at home, there's a good chance that your IT department knows exactly what you are doing. And eventually your bosses probably will, too.

Disadvantages of Online Porn

There are some pitfalls related to online porn that you need to keep in mind. A few areas of concern include the following.

Charges and Fees

Just as people who called 900 numbers would often get shockingly high phone bills, people who view online porn can also run into unexpected charges. Watch out for sites that lure you in with limited free offerings but then require you to pay a fee for the full inventory. Many sites also give you a brief trial period but then automatically charge your credit card if you don't cancel. Your best bet is to never enter your credit card information on any online adult site. If you really feel the need to access paid material, limit yourself to one reputable site—and be sure to keep a close watch on your credit card statements. Sites affiliated with well-known adult magazines, X-rated movie companies, or adult toy shops are usually among the safest and most reputable choices.

Viruses and Other Computer Problems

Porn sites are notorious for being loaded with viruses, spyware, and other stuff that can really mess up your computer. Make sure you have a good anti-virus program installed and steer clear of any sites that look the least bit suspicious.

Accidental Discoveries

Unethical websites will often arrange it so their sites show up on Internet searches for relatively benign search words. For example, if you search for "French kissing," some of the search results may actually be for sites involving group sex or bondage. (As any web-savvy parent can attest after her child made a shocking discovery, even a search for something totally unrelated to sex can sometimes lead to porn. For example, a search for Santa Claus could turn up X-rated pictures of a naked guy in a Santa hat getting it on with a group of female elves.)

No matter how careful you are, it's possible that you will view something way more graphic than you had intended. Be prepared for that possibility, and be ready to close your browser window quickly if you get an unpleasant surprise.

Risk of Addiction

Because online porn is so plentiful and easily accessible, many people find it very addictive. It's becoming increasingly common for people to spend hours looking at online porn, often hiding the activity from their spouses or partners. The risk of addiction can be very harmful to a relationship because a compulsion to constantly view online porn affects not only the addicted person, but also her partner. The addicted person may spend an excessive amount of time online, neglecting her relationship with her partner (and other important things in her life). She also may become so infatuated with online sexual material that her real-life sex life suffers, possibly even ceasing altogether.

Porn addiction can be a serious problem. Treatment can help, so look into programs like those offered through the Sexual Recovery Institute (*www.sexualrecovery.com*) or find a treatment center at a clearinghouse like Recovery Connection (*www.recoveryconnection.org*).

You should also get into the habit of clearing your computer's cookies and history after each online porn viewing session, especially if other people ever use your computer. Otherwise, an unsuspecting friend or family member may get a shocking surprise the next time they log on.

Video Cameras and Web Cams

Video cameras—both the traditional kind and the web cam variety—can be a relatively easy way to add some excitement to your sex life. Most cameras are very easy to use and are available in affordable models.

Video Cameras

Video cameras have been around for quite a while, and people have probably been using them for sexual purposes almost as long. Many couples find it exciting to videotape their sexual exploits and watch them later. Sometimes one partner will play the role of cameraman while the other is the star, and then reverse roles.

It can indeed be exciting to watch yourself and your partner perform sexual acts on video. It can be just like watching an X-rated movie, only you and your partners are the stars.

However, as many people know, there have been numerous cases in which someone was horrified to discover a private video fell into the wrong hands. Many modern cameras actually make digital recordings, making it extremely simple for someone to upload and quickly distribute footage online.

Web Cams

A web cam is a camera used with a computer. It may either be built into the computer or added on as a separate external element. Either way, the recording process is generally simple. You simply aim the web cam at whatever you want to record, push a button on the computer, and the footage is either stored on your computer or broadcast instantly online.

Web cams are a popular way for friends, relatives, and couples to add a personal face to their online chats. Some couples use it to share racy or intimate footage with each other while exchanging sexual messages online. Or one or both partners could post explicit footage online.

As with other type of pictures and video footage, web cam footage can easily be copied and broadcast online. Remember, once you post something on the Internet, you lose control over where it goes and who sees it.

Racy E-mails and Text Messages

While most people who engage in cybersex prefer the immediate response capabilities of instant messaging or chat programs, you may not always have access to those options. In that case, you might want to send your sexy messages via e-mail or text.

E-mail

As cybersex options go, e-mail is probably considered the most basic. Almost anyone who uses a computer knows how to send an e-mail message, so it's very simple. On the downside, there's a lag in response time. Even if the recipient types a reply immediately, it may take a while for the message to appear in your inbox. This constant delay can make it tough to conduct a steamy X-rated exchange without destroying the mood.

Keep in mind that anything you send via e-mail or text messaging can easily be forwarded to someone else without your knowledge. Be sure to only send racy messages to someone you trust completely, and remind them to delete the messages after viewing them.

Text Messages

Text messaging is extremely popular right now—and, as a result, so is sending sexual text messages. The process of sending sex-related text messages has become known as *sexting*, especially when done among teens.

ESSENTIAL

You should only engage in racy text messaging if your phone (and your partner's) is off-limits to other people. If someone else uses your phone, you don't want them accidentally getting a peek at your private exchange. Regardless, it's a good idea to delete all remnants of your sex talk as soon as possible.

Text messaging is easy and convenient. Nearly all newer cell phones have texting capabilities. There can also be an element of naughtiness and secrecy, such as if your partner receives an erotic text message from you while she is in a business meeting. (Bonus: If your partner's phone is set on vibrate, your message can provide her with an added little secret thrill.) To avoid typing overly lengthy messages, come up with your own secret sexy shorthand—and be creative, so you can exchange texts that only the two of you will understand.

As with e-mail and instant messaging, most text messaging services also allow you to attach images (and perhaps even video clips).

High-Tech Sex Toys

If you haven't checked out the latest sex toys in a while, you might be a little bit shocked at the modern options available now. While there are still plenty of standard battery-operated models, there are also many types of sex toys that have lots of fancy bells and whistles. For example, there are vibrators with a dozen or so different speeds and other settings, sex toys that are meant for both partners to use at once, and sex toys that come equipped with sound effects—you name it, it's probably already out there.

Here are a few of the newest high-tech sexual accessories:

- Vibrating underwear that comes with a remote control, so one partner can give the other a surprise "zap" at unexpected times.
- Taking that one step further, there are vibrators that operate by wireless remote control.

- A battery-operated vibrating glove has tiny vibrating pads in the fingers, adding a whole array of new sensations during manual stimulation.
- There's also an online company that sells a large padded seat with a built in dildo—the device plugs into an electrical outlet and rocks and vibrates as the woman straddles it.

Like other sexual options, these are all simply a matter of taste and preference. Some people find sex toys with fancy extras to be exciting, while others find them distracting, annoying, or even scary. If you aren't sure how you feel about these high-tech toys, it's smart to try something relatively mild (and not too challenging to operate) and then work your way up to something fancier as your comfort level allows.

CHAPTER 22

For the Really Daring

People have lots of different bedroom personalities, especially when it comes to how bold and daring they are willing to be. For some people, simply trying a new position is adventurous enough. For others, things can get stale quickly if they aren't constantly shaking things up in the bedroom. The majority of people fall somewhere in between. It's all a matter of finding your own comfort zone, figuring out your boundaries and deciding when and if you are willing to explore new territory. The activities in this chapter admittedly aren't for everyone, but the most daring among you might be eager to try one or two of them at least once.

Exhibitionism

Even if they won't admit it, many people get a thrill out of knowing someone is watching them when they are naked or partially undressed and in a "private" moment. (Of course, this assumes that you are aware you are being watched and are okay with it. This is totally different from being the victim of a peeping Tom, which most people find disturbing and not the least bit sexy—not to mention illegal.)

As an exhibitionist, you are mainly enjoying the fact that you know the person (or people) watching you finds you and your activities sexy and exciting. You have his undivided attention, and he is totally captivated by your every move. You can get a strange sense of power by knowing you have this effect on someone else.

Remember, just because you like someone watching you in an intimate moment doesn't necessarily mean you want to have an intimate moment with him. Most exhibitionists like to keep their show a strictly one-sided performance. Some people who engage in a swinging or open lifestyle do take their exhibitionism to the next level and invite their audience to join in. But it's very possible to be an exhibitionist and still be in a faithful, monogamous relationship.

Solo Exhibitionism

The majority of people who engage in exhibitionism do it alone, and in a passive way—often making it seem accidental. For example, they will get undressed in front of a window and "forget" to close the drapes. If you are very creative, you may also be able to arrange it so that someone spots you masturbating, but it will take a little bit of thought to figure out how to manage this.

This type of thing can be a win-win situation: the performer gets to play the exhibitionist, while the person watching gets to engage in a voyeuristic thrill, believing they got a glimpse of something they weren't supposed to see. Whether to let on that you are aware you are being watched is up to you.

Keep in mind, though, that there's a fine line between exhibitionism and indecent exposure. You should try to be reasonably certain that your observer wants to see your "show." If there's any doubt, stick to relatively tame tactics, such as showing an "accidental" fleeting glance of your lingerie or a bare thigh. And, of course, you should never expose too much skin in any environment where a child may be watching.

ESSENTIAL

In 2009, the Standard Hotel opened in Manhattan, boasting floor-to-ceiling windows and a stellar view of the High Line Park below. But the people in the park got just as good a view of the antics of naked hotel guests. The hotel eventually issued a statement saying it would "remind guests of the transparency of the windows."

Joint Exhibitionism

If your partner is also an exhibitionist (or secretly wants to be), the two of you may find it exciting to make love while someone else watches. Again, it's possible to do this in a passive way, simply by having sex in front of a window—or, if you are really daring, outside—so it's likely that someone else will spot you.

Another option: You could research sex clubs or swinger get-togethers. Be sure you are clear on the rules, though. Some clubs do allow couples to be exhibitionists without engaging in sexual contact with their audience, while at other clubs this is considered rude or selfish. If it is allowed, there is probably some kind of sign or code you must use so that others know they can watch but can't touch.

Two-Way Exhibitionism

An exciting way to take exhibitionism to the next level is to engage in a two-way show. This is where your audience knows you are aware of their presence and decides to return the favor and put on a show for you. As a result, you each get to be both voyeurs and exhibitionists. For some people, this adds an extra thrill, while others prefer the one-sided "accidental" exhibitionism because they don't feel the pressure to reciprocate or even acknowledge the other person's presence. Keep in mind that by acknowledging the other person's attention and actively interacting with them (even from a distance), you increase the odds that they will want to make contact with you—which could be an unwelcome (and possibly unsafe) move.

ALERT

Be warned: Your partner may not be happy to discover that you are putting on a sexy show for someone else. This is especially true if you are engaging in a two-way exhibitionism situation. This is a very individual thing, though. Some partners may find it exciting and may even be eager to join you in your exhibitionist activities.

Threesomes

Though they may be reluctant to admit it (even to themselves), many people find the thought of a threesome to be exciting and sexy. The idea of bringing another person into the bedroom can be both naughty and thrilling—not to mention, there would be another set of hands (and other body parts), which makes all sorts of new positions and anatomical arrangements possible. But taking it from fantasy to reality is a big step. If you are even contemplating engaging in a threesome, you should take plenty of time to think it through carefully first.

While some couples swear that engaging in one or more threesomes spiced up their sex lives immensely, others regret having tried a threesome and perhaps even cite the experience as a fatal blow to their relationship. It's common for feelings of jealousy or insecurity to come into play, and at least one partner can often end up wishing he had never participated in a threesome at all.

This is something you and your partner should definitely discuss in depth beforehand. If you do decide to forge ahead, establish some ground rules you both find agreeable—especially when it comes to selecting the third member of your threesome.

The Gender Ratio of Your Threesome

You and your partner may have both expressed an interest in a threesome, but further discussion may reveal you each have a much different vision of what that threesome might look like. For example, many men are turned on by the idea of sex with two women but may be turned off by a threesome featuring another guy. On the other hand, a woman might be excited at the thought at having two men—but then again, she might be curious about what it would be like to have another woman join her and her partner in bed.

Sometimes, a person is okay with watching his partner play with someone else, but wants to remain a spectator and doesn't want to engage with the third party. Or, it may be the opposite—he may want to engage in sexual activities with the third party while his partner just watches or interacts only with him, not touching the third party.

ESSENTIAL

It is common for the member of a couple who is the same gender as the potential third party to have mixed feelings about the idea. While he may be aroused by the thought, he may also fear being seen as a homosexual. A frank discussion about experimentation versus sexual orientation might be helpful in this situation.

There's no one-size-fits-all arrangement that works for everyone. The important thing is to hash this out with your partner right from the start to avoid any conflicts or unpleasant surprises later.

Before you embark on a threesome, be prepared for the possibility that things may not go as you planned, especially when it comes to the ground rules you've established with your partner. No matter how firmly you or your partner swear you will or won't do a certain thing, that resolve may go out the window once clothes start coming off. That's a risk you take in this situation.

Selecting Your Third Party

Once you and your partner decide you would like to try a threesome, there is a practical matter to consider. That is, who will be the third member of your little intimate group? This can be tricky and challenging. After all, it's not like you can just call up your neighbor and ask if he would like to come over and join the two of you in a sex romp. (Unless of course you have an unusually close relationship with your neighbor.)

ESSENTIAL

Whenever you and/or your partner are engaging in any kind of intimate acts with someone new, you should always practice safe sex. While it is great to ask the other person about her sexual history, she may not always be totally honest. Ideally, all parties involved should get tested for sexual transmitted diseases beforehand.

When it comes to selecting a third party, there are basically two main schools of thought. Some couples prefer to select a stranger who they will never see again. They may put this stranger though some kind of screening process beforehand—say, by making initial contact through a personal ad or online venue—so they can ensure there is a good match. This also gives you an opportunity to establish your requirements (for example, the drug and disease free notation is a common screening criteria). Swinger clubs can also be a good tool for making this sort of connection, because they often establish ground rules that all parties must agree to, and they also often offer some kind of host location, which provides at least a small sense of security.

On the other hand, there are couples who prefer to pick someone with whom they already have an existing relationship, thus turning a platonic friend into a friend with benefits. The advantage here is that this person is someone with whom the couple already has a bond of friendship and trust. It is also likely that they all know each other's sexual history already, which may make everyone feel safer and more comfortable.

ESSENTIAL

When first approaching a friend about a threesome, many couples will initially wait for an opportunity when they and the friend are relaxed and enjoying a few drinks. They will then broach the subject in a seemingly joking manner, just to see how the person reacts. Should that person not be receptive to the idea, they can always claim to have been joking (or tipsy).

It can be tricky (not to mention awkward) to approach a potential third party for your threesome. The best advice comes from people who have been there and done that. Check out the forums at swinger sites like *www.swingersboard.com* where people share stories about approach methods they have tried.

There's a downside to inviting someone you know into your bedroom. Should things go badly, you will probably still have to face this person on a regular basis, which could make for some uncomfortable and awkward moments. Also, having a threesome with a friend or acquaintance makes it more likely that other people in your social circle will find out about your activities.

The Aftermath

Here is a word of warning for couples who may be contemplating or planning a threesome. Many couples who do take the plunge and engage in a threesome find they have some serious issues to contend with afterward. Often, at least one partner will have gotten hooked and will decide this is something they want to do again—perhaps on a regular basis. This can be a problem if the other partner doesn't feel the same way. If the gung-ho partner really pushes for a repeat, the other person may start to feel insecure, wondering if he alone is no longer enough to satisfy his partner.

While this is something you should anticipate and discuss beforehand, this is a situation where you often don't know how you will feel until you are actually in that position. Just be prepared for this possibility, and know that it could require some serious discussions between you and your partner.

Group Sex and Swinging

Perhaps you and your partner have tried a threesome, enjoyed it—and want something even more exciting. Or maybe you want to just skip the threesome and dive right into more adventurous territory. You may be contemplating group sex.

Many of the same issues and warnings mentioned in the section on threesomes also apply here. One of the advantages touted by couples who prefer group sex to threesomes: With more parties involved, it is less likely that one partner will end up feeling like a neglected third wheel, as can sometimes happen with a threesome.

Generally, the easiest way to get into a group sex situation is by swinging. *Swinging*—or *the lifestyle*, as it is often called by participants—can take many forms. Some swingers' groups are organized and formal, involving membership fees, rules, and so on. Others are more informal, often involving people who meet via online message boards or chat lists.

FACT

Swinging clubs often have a set of rules and etiquette (these may be written, or may just be assumed as understood). The members and leaders of these groups take these rules very seriously. Before attending any events or joining any activities, be sure you understand and are okay with the rules of that particular group.

The route you choose is totally up to you and your partner. One rule of thumb: The more hoops you need to jump through, the higher a level of security and discretion you can usually expect.

S&M/Bondage

Many couples enjoy bondage or S&M types of sexual play, although this is a broad category that can really run the gamut from mild to wild. For some, it may simply mean using a paddle for some light spanking or furry handcuffs for harmless restraints. Other couples are into more hardcore types of activities: leashes or collars and serious restraints, hot wax, whips, etc. The important thing is to make sure you and your partner are both comfortable with the choice of S&M tactics.

When engaging in S&M activities, many couples find it important to have a safe word, which would signal that they want to stop immediately. This word should be something obscure, as opposed to a common word like "No!" which people often blurt out instinctively in the heat of passion. Both partners must respect this rule and agree to abide by the signal word.

It is not uncommon for people to be more turned on by the idea of being tied up, punished, or whipped than they are by the actual reality. Often, one or both partners will realize these S&M tactics may be more painful and/or embarrassing than they had expected. So it's a good idea to start on the mild end of the spectrum—say, by tying each other up with scarves or engaging in light spanking—and slowly working your way up to more daring stuff if you feel comfortable.

If you are really serious about pursuing your S&M fantasies, you may even want to try to find a dominatrix in your area. These are women who specialize in performing dominating—and sometimes abusive—techniques in order to stimulate sexual arousal in their clients. (They generally don't actually have sex with clients, though.) Some even provide instructional services, where they will teach one person how to better employ domination techniques with a submissive partner.

Risky Behavior

There are some sex-related activities that are for the truly fearless (or the truly reckless, depending on whom you ask). Here's a list of a few of them.

- Having sex in your parents' house, a cemetery, the office, or some other place that most people consider off-limits or too risky.
- Having sex in a very public location where you are certain to be caught (and perhaps even arrested).
- Getting a piercing or tattoo in a very private place, perhaps at the same time as your partner.
- Having unprotected sex with a person or persons whose history you don't know.
- Taking your clothes off and putting on a sexy performance in public, such as at amateur night at a local strip club.
- Making your own amateur adult video and uploading it to a porn site online.

Remember, if you decide to try any of these, you do so at your own risk.

APPENDIX

Resources

Hotlines

National STD Hotline: 1-800-227-8922

National AIDS Hotline: 1-800-342-2437

Note: these two hotlines recently formed a partnership, and are now both under the umbrella of the National CDC STD and AIDS Hotline program. Both numbers are still in effect, and you can also get information at the program's website at *www.doe.in.gov/sservices/hivaids_cdchotline.html.*

Further Reading

Anand, Margot. *The Art of Sexual Ecstasy.* (Los Angeles: Jeremy P. Tarcher, 1989).

Berman, Jennifer, M.D., and Laura Berman, Ph.D. *For Women Only: A Revolutionary Guide to Overcoming Sexual Dysfunction and Reclaiming Your Sex Life.* (New York: Henry Holt & Company, 2001).

Campbell, Susan M. *The Couple's Journey: Intimacy as a Path to Wholeness.* (San Luis Obispo, CA: Impact Publishers, 1980).

Camphausen, Rufus C. *The Encyclopedia of Sacred Sexuality.* (Rochester, VT: Inner Traditions, 1999).

Chia, Mantak and Maneewan Chia, *Healing Love Through the Tao: Cultivating Female Sexual Energy,* (Huntington, NY: Healing Tao Books, 1986; reissued, 1991).

Chia, Mantak and Douglas Abrams. *The Multi-Orgasmic Man.* (San Francisco: HarperCollins, 1997).

Dempsey, Bobbi. *1,001 Sexcapades to Do If You Dare* (Avon, MA: Adams Media, 2008).

Dempsey, Bobbi. *The Everything Tantric Sex Book* (Avon, MA: Adams Media, 2007).

Douglas, Nik and Penny Slinger. *Sexual Secrets: The Alchemy of Ecstasy.* (Rochester, VT: Inner Traditions, 1979; reprint, 1999).

Meletis, Chris D. *Better Sex Naturally: Herbs and Other Supplements That Can Jump Start Your Sex Life.* (New York: Chrysalis Books, 2000).

Muir, Charles and Caroline Muir. *Tantra: The Art of Conscious Loving.* (San Francisco: Mercury House, Inc., 1989).

Ramsdale, David and Ellen Ramsdale. *Sexual Energy Ecstasy: A Practical Guide to Lovemaking Secrets of the East and West.* (Playa Del Rey, CA: Peak Skill Publishing, 1991; reprint, New York: Bantam Doubleday, 1993).

Stubbs, Kenneth Ray, Ph.D. *The Essential Tantra: A Modern Guide to Sacred Sexuality.* (New York: Jeremy P. Tarcher, 2000).

Zilbergeld, Bernie, Ph.D. *The New Male Sexuality.* (New York: Bantam Books, 1999).

INDEX

Find out Everything on Anything
at everything.com!

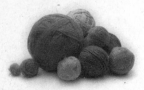

The new **Everything.com** has answers to your questions on just about everything! Based on the bestselling Everything book series, the **Everything.com** community provides a unique connection between members and experts in a variety of fields. Since 1996, Everything experts have helped millions of readers learn something new in an easy-to-understand, accessible, and fun way. And now Everything advice and know-how is available online.

At **Everything.com** you can explore thousands of articles on hundreds of topics—from starting your own business and personal finance to health-care advice and help with parenting, cooking, learning a new language, and more. And you also can:

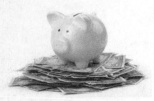

- **Share advice**
- **Rate articles**
- **Submit articles**
- **Sign up for our Everything.com newsletters to stay informed of the latest articles, areas of interest, exciting sweepstakes, and more!**

Visit **Everything.com** where you'll find the broadest range and most authoritative content available online!

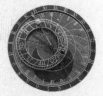

31901050402363